W9-CMQ-462

Advance Acclaim

"How does exercise potentially prevent Alzheimer's disease? What type of memory problems should concern us as we age? What memory strategies actually work? Dr. Randolph has created an accessible, practical guide to improving brain health. Quizzes, case examples, myth-busting, and a user-friendly dive into relevant neuroscience make this an enjoyable, life-altering read."

—**Karen Postal, Ph.D., ABPP**, Neuropsychologist, Clinical Instructor, Harvard Medical School

"This book provides everything you need to know about preserving cognitive capacity as you age. Dr. Randolph has reviewed massive amounts of relevant research, translated it into a language everyone can understand, and extracted the important take-aways that allow the reader to convert words into action. I found particularly helpful the last chapter that summarizes the science of habit formation. This book does not over-promise (a pet peeve of mine when I look at self-help books), but gives the reader a blueprint for how to go about making lifestyle changes that can have a significant impact on brain health."

—**Peg Dawson, Ed.D.**, Staff Psychologist, Seacoast Mental Health Center, Portsmouth, NH, co-author of numerous books on executive skills, including *The Smart but Scattered Guide to Success: How to Use Your Brain's Executive Skills to Keep Up, Stay Calm, and Get Organized at Work and at Home*

The Brain Health Book

The Brain
Health Book

USING THE POWER OF
NEUROSCIENCE TO IMPROVE
YOUR LIFE

JOHN RANDOLPH

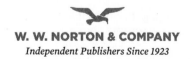

W. W. NORTON & COMPANY
Independent Publishers Since 1923

Important Note: *The Brain Health Book* is intended to provide general information on the subject of brain health. It is not a substitute for professional diagnosis of or treatment for cognitive impairment. If you are experiencing memory or other cognitive loss, see a healthcare provider who specializes in those areas. Also see your doctor or other healthcare provider before you undertake a new exercise program and before you add new foods to your diet, if you have or may have allergies.

For information about permission to reproduce selections from this book, write to Permissions, W. W. Norton & Company, Inc., 500 Fifth Avenue, New York, NY 10110

For information about special discounts for bulk purchases, please contact W. W. Norton Special Sales at specialsales@wwnorton.com or 800-233-4830

Manufacturing by Lake Book Manufacturing, Inc.
Production manager: Katelyn MacKenzie

Library of Congress Cataloging-in-Publication Data

Names: Randolph, John J., author.
Title: The brain health book : using the power of neuroscience to improve your life / John Randolph.
Description: First edition. | New York : W.W. Norton & Company, [2020] | Includes bibliographical references and index.
Identifiers: LCCN 2019014870 | ISBN 9780393712872 (hardcover)
Subjects: LCSH: Brain—Popular works. | Neurophysiology—Popular works.
Classification: LCC QP376 .R36 2020 | DDC 612.8/2—dc23
LC record available at https://lccn.loc.gov/2019014870

W. W. Norton & Company, Inc., 500 Fifth Avenue, New York, N.Y. 10110
www.wwnorton.com

W. W. Norton & Company Ltd., 15 Carlisle Street, London W1D 3BS

1 2 3 4 5 6 7 8 9 0

For Kaia

CONTENTS

PREFACE

INFORMATION ABOUT THE BRAIN—AND HOW TO potentially improve its many functions—has become increasingly available in popular culture. Newspaper articles, online sources, and talk show hosts are often eager to tout the findings from one-off studies that purportedly clarify how the brain works or how it can work better. Commercials and junk e-mails praise the benefits of supplements or other products that are supposed to magically transform the brain's inner workings. But what actually helps, and what's hype? Is there compelling science out there that can be translated and used to inform our decisions, strategies, and lifestyle choices?

In the 2000s, I started taking more notice of the science of brain health. I also wondered why this topic was not being discussed more frequently in my neuropsychology circles or in academic journals. Being a neuropsychologist—a clinical psychologist specializing in brain–behavior relationships— I was much more aware of how to document and diagnose cognitive disorders than how to promote better thinking skills. Throughout my training, I heard repeatedly that once the brain was injured, diseased, aging, or otherwise not working properly, there simply wasn't much we could do about it. I never wanted to believe this.

As I continued to dive into research on brain wellness, I thought it would be useful to summarize some of it for my colleagues at an upcoming meeting. I gave a presentation on the topic and thought perhaps that would be it. Fate then intervened in the form of a publisher who had heard about my seminar and suggested that I consider writing a related book for a professional audience. I accepted this offer and enjoyed the labors and rewards of writing and editing a reference on brain health for people in my field.

During that process, I kept coming back to the idea that people outside my small professional zone would probably be interested in a book that considered the science of brain health. It seemed that it might be useful to translate the research for folks who were curious about neuroscience, neuropsychology, brain health, and related fields, but who hadn't necessarily been educated in those areas. Perhaps consider the science in a way that wouldn't go too far into the weeds but nevertheless clarified some brain-related ideas and terms we might hear in the media. Maybe share some of my own excitement related to recent developments in neuroscience—like our ability to grow neurons by exercising, a concept foreign to essentially all medical professionals and researchers until fairly recently—and help clarify practical applications for our daily lives.

This is that book. I earnestly hope that you enjoy it. I also hope that you become fascinated and inspired by the cutting-edge neuroscience and behavioral research discussed here that is transforming our ability to make our brains healthier. Of course, science should not be kept in a vacuum: you can apply what's reviewed here immediately to potentially improve your own brain functioning, and, ultimately, your life. I've also included some case composites throughout the book that detail how lifestyle choices have positively impacted cognitive skills in people I've worked with. Incidentally, if you're interested in getting into the scientific details, there are plenty of references to academic papers at the back of the book that represent some of the most innovative brain health studies. You're also welcome to not worry about any of that for now.

Either way, I encourage you to get comfortable, read through some or all of the chapters based on your interests, and appreciate that most of what we know of that helps the brain is free or inexpensive, fun, emotionally enriching, and stimulating (not to mention tasty). Your brain will thank you for it.

The Brain Health Book

PART I

Introduction to Your Brain and How It Works

1

The Four Domains of Brain Health

WHEN WE THINK ABOUT *HEALTH*, WE DEFINE IT IN a number of ways. Physical health refers to our ability to stay free of illness or to recover quickly when we get sick. Cardiovascular health relates to how well our heart and blood vessels are working. Mental health can refer to many things, but usually this is discussed in the context of how we regulate our emotions and manage stress. We all strive to live in ways that maximize our health, although this is certainly easier said than done.

This book focuses on the type of health that I consider "the elephant in the room": brain health, also known as cognitive health. **All other aspects of health fundamentally depend on brain and cognitive health.** The better we make decisions, remember new information, concentrate on tasks, and process information efficiently, the more likely our body will be firing on all cylinders. Your brain's ability to function at its highest level is critically important regardless of whether you're in school, working, raising a family, or retired.

You've probably seen references to brain wellness or cognitive health in lots of places. Your e-mail inbox may have been inundated with messages touting the benefits of supplements you may or may not have heard of. Perhaps you've watched infomercials on TV describing products or programs guaranteed to improve your memory in a short period of time. The supposed benefits of computerized "brain games" are trumpeted broadly. There are also a number of books on the topic of brain health; some have merit, while others might function best as kindling for a holiday fire.

This book isn't promoting a quick fix related to improving how your brain works. Think about it: if we were able to change our brains over a short period of time with a magic pill or strategy, wouldn't we all be doing this already? The brain has evolved to its current incredible state over hundreds of thousands of years. A marketing pitch that claims to change it meaningfully in a few days or weeks is simply, as my grandmother used to say, "hogwash."

That being said, there is a large body of scientific research that clarifies what we can do, over time, to help our brains work more efficiently, encode new information more effectively, and concentrate more precisely on the task at hand. **The focus of this book is on translating the science of brain and cognitive health into a program you can use.** We will consider a variety of strategies, lifestyle activities, dietary choices, and other factors that are known to promote the brain's ability to function well. We will also discuss ways to learn positive, brain-healthy habits one step at a time and get around the barriers that may have interfered with developing these habits in the past. Changing our behavior is hard. But developing new routines and ways of living is doable, particularly when done using incremental steps over time— and when we take some related tips from science.

Here's how this book is organized. The first three chapters will provide some background information about neuroscience, cognitive health, and how the brain works. Later in this chapter, I'll introduce what I consider to be a useful and easily remembered model of brain and cognitive health. We'll refer to this model throughout the book as a broad perspective on how we can think about positive strategies and lifestyle changes known to nurture and improve the brain.

Beginning with Chapter 4, you'll see a consistent three-part structure in the chapters. I'll start each chapter with a section called "The Background Science." This is where I'll summarize recent and past research that's been done on a given topic, say, benefits of exercise for the brain or how nutrition affects our thinking skills. This section will help clarify the importance of a topic as it relates to the brain so that you'll understand why the topic has been included in the book. In case you're interested in learning more, there are references to important studies in the chapter notes section at the end of the book.

A review of the science will set up the next section of each chapter, "The Bottom Line." As you might have guessed, "The Bottom Line" will be a brief summary of key scientific findings and related applications that you can refer to at any time as a quick refresher.

The final section of each chapter is "The Brass Tacks." This section will help you put everything together and do some personal strategic planning to move you in the direction you want to go. It will be laid out in a worksheet format to help you create your own blueprint for developing brain-boosting habits. You'll see spaces where you can record your current level of activity, clarify barriers that have gotten in the way in the past (or might in the future), and set near-term and more distant goals for increasing that activity over time. This sort of strategic planning can be very powerful in effecting change. We know that monitoring our own behavior is one of the best ways not only to improve awareness of what our tendencies are but also to make changes we want (or need) to make.

It's important to point out that this book is designed so that the reader can begin any section or chapter at any time. Don't feel compelled to read chapters in order, from start to finish; perhaps the chapter on exercise is of particular interest, or maybe you'd like to start with the content related to social activity and the brain. There are many different ways to promote brain and cognitive health, and you should take a look at what seems to be most relevant for you as you strive to make positive lifestyle changes.

MYTHS AND MISCONCEPTIONS
ABOUT THE BRAIN

Sometimes in popular culture, we hear things about how the brain works from the news, people we know, and heathcare professionals. It's remarkable how some of this information can be repeated again and again, even if there really isn't scientific evidence supporting it. **Let's review and critique a few common beliefs (or misconceptions):**

- Significant memory loss is a natural part of the aging process.

Don't believe this one for a second. This is one of the biggest misconceptions about the aging process: that no matter what, our brains will atrophy and we'll develop Alzheimer's disease or another form of dementia. In fact, until we get into our nineties, most of us will not experience significant memory or other cognitive impairment. Even then, over 50% of people remain dementia free for most of that decade. Further, we know that some people have brains that age remarkably well—a group of elders who researchers call "Superagers"—and show very few if any brain-related changes even compared to people 30 years younger. They also show memory abilities that rival those of middle-aged adults. The bottom line is that memory impairment is definitely not part of the typical aging process for most of us.

- Our lifestyle activities in midlife don't have much of an impact on our memory and other thinking skills later in life.

If you thought this was true, you probably wouldn't be reading this book. We're learning more and more about how our activity levels, diet, and overall interest or disinterest in wellness affect how cognitively healthy we are in the future. For example, we know that higher physical fitness in midlife is linked to better brain health 20+ years later. Throughout this book, we'll discuss how engaging in different lifestyle activities will increase the chances of having a better-looking and better-working brain down the road.

- Positive changes in the brain occur throughout life.

Years ago, neurologists thought that the brain was essentially set in stone beginning fairly early in life. Once the brain had gone through its initial development, it simply was done growing. The only changes thought to occur at that point were negative ones: loss of neurons, atrophy of the cerebral cortex, and depleted brain chemicals or neurotransmitters. Now we know the story is nowhere near that bleak. In fact, it's almost the opposite: the brain continues to grow and adapt throughout life, into our eighties and beyond. I was struck by a study a few years ago that found that sedentary individuals in their eighties who began an exercise program experienced significant (and positive) changes in the connections between multiple brain regions. Becoming more active and making wellness-oriented lifestyle choices—at any point in life—will inevitably fine-tune the brain.

Along these lines, studies show that people who stay mentally or physically engaged experience growth in different parts of the brain—evidence of new neurons or better connections between existing neurons—and perform better on standardized cognitive tests. This refers to what we call *plasticity*: the ability of the brain to change, adapt, and grow over time in positive ways.

- Forgetting something you recently learned or used to know is an early sign of dementia.

When I see patients for neuropsychological evaluations, this is often their greatest fear. They may have recently met someone whose name they can no longer recall or forgotten an appointment that had been scheduled a few months ago. Perhaps they can't remember the name of a street they used to drive on years back. One of the fundamental tenets of brain functioning is this: we actually forget lots of things, and that's okay. Can you name what you had for dinner four nights ago? Can you remember the name of someone you briefly met for the first time at a concert last month? Simply put, when we are exposed to new information, some of it sticks (and we'll talk later about how to improve this process), and some of it doesn't.

Dementia is a different animal. Not remembering where you parked your car at a shopping mall is relatively common. Forgetting whether you drove, took the bus, or rode in a taxi to the mall is more troubling. Another example: we all misplace our keys from time to time, but few of us mistakenly put our keys in the freezer when we get home. If you're truly concerned about cognitive changes, and others who know you are too, it might be a good time to see a neuropsychologist or neurologist for an evaluation. That being said, it's important to note that many people experience memory and other cognitive lapses because of stress, sleep problems, chronic pain, inattention, and other factors that probably don't reflect a brain-related disorder per se.

- Medications that treat memory problems are very effective.

Unfortunately, at this point, this is a misconception. We have a few medications that improve daily functioning for some people, but the gains are usually minor and short lived. There simply is no silver-bullet medication or supplement that returns one's memory to where it once was. Don't believe the marketing hype of the latest "brain health supplement" you hear about on TV or elsewhere. Fortunately, we do know that social engagement, exercise, mental stimulation, and other lifestyle choices are associated with better cognitive skills and may even prevent dementia in some people.

- If it's going to affect us, Alzheimer's disease usually starts in our forties or fifties.

The earliest that Alzheimer's disease begins to affect most people is in their mid to late sixties, although mild cognitive impairment—memory or other cognitive difficulties that do not cause significant problems in daily life—can begin somewhat earlier. There is a very rare form of early-onset Alzheimer's disease that can occur in midlife, but the vast majority of Alzheimer's cases start after age 65.

- Once your memory has begun to decline, there's nothing you can do about it.

Also untrue. Most of us experience subtle changes to our thinking skills as we get older, beginning sometime in middle age. Our life experiences, well-established professional skills, and ability to proceed through life more efficiently than when we were younger can all provide a buffer against those mild changes. But we also know that individuals who age the best—cognitively and physically—are the ones who stay the most active. The science also indicates that even individuals with cognitive impairment, including those with dementia, can enhance their brain skills through exercise and other types of activity.

- We only use 10% of our brains.

Simply put, if this were accurate, brain scans such as brain magnetic resonance imaging (brain MRI) would show large areas of dead tissue. While it may be the case that people use their brains differently, unless you have a neurologic disorder such as stroke or dementia, you're generally using all of your brain in different ways throughout the day (and night).

THE C.A.P.E.ˢᴹ MODEL OF BRAIN HEALTH

Throughout this book, we'll use an easy-to-remember model—the C.A.P.E. model—as a reference for four key domains that are linked to better brain and cognitive health. C.A.P.E. is an acronym that stands for the following:

- Cognitive strategies
- Activity engagement
- Prevention of cognitive problems
- Education about the brain

Because I'm a big fan of learning information in different ways, we can also consider this model in graphical form (Figure 1.1).

Let's discuss the four parts of the model. The "C" of the C.A.P.E. model, *cognitive strategies*, refers to different techniques we can use to enhance our ability to remember, organize, and manage information in daily life. Some people use their cell phone calendars to record and later

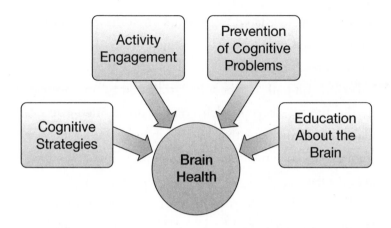

FIGURE 1.1 C.A.P.E.^{SM} Model of Brain Health

remind them of upcoming appointments; others prefer paper-based organizers. So-called sticky notes are a great way to clarify tasks that need to be completed in the near future (or decorate the perimeter of our computer monitors at work). Reminders from kitchen timers can help us remember to turn off the stove or to take a mid-day medication dose. These are all examples of cognitive strategies, specifically what we call *external strategies*—strategies that are external to or outside of us. Any sort of physical aid used to help us manage the daily flow of information would fall into this category.

Another (often complementary) type of strategy is the *internal strategy*—a technique we generate mentally to facilitate learning, recall, or other cognitive processing. Susan was a patient of mine who regularly used a great internal strategy: creating stories with information she wanted to

learn and retrieve later. Despite having some memory problems, she was able to craft some great tales, including one
where cereal boxes walked to the produce section to attend
a tomato and bell pepper soirée, followed by an after party
in the freezer section with some truly chilled-out Lean
Cuisines—funny, creative, and much better (at least for her)
than trying to remember a boring and somewhat random
grocery list.

The C.A.P.E. model itself is an example of an internal
strategy; an acronym like C.A.P.E. serves as a quick reference to the broader process of helping our brains work
better. We'll talk much more about cognitive strategies in
Chapter 4.

The "A" of the C.A.P.E. model refers to *activity*, more
specifically, engagement in lifestyle activities. What types of
activities, you ask? There are three primary types of activity
that have been researched extensively and are linked to better
brain functioning. The most science to date has been devoted
to the first type of activity referenced by the C.A.P.E. model:
physical activity. The benefits of exercise on the brain have
received quite a bit of press, and you may have seen some
related stories in your local newspaper, online, or on TV.
The research points almost entirely in the same direction:
the more fit and physically active you are, the better your
brain will work, and the more robust your processing speed,
memory, and other cognitive skills will likely be.

There's also evidence that people who exercise regularly
are less prone to developing cognitive impairment later in

life, including some forms of dementia. And if you're reading this book in midlife, keep in mind that physical fitness in our forties and fifties is strongly associated with our cognitive health in older age. Fundamentally, exercise may be the best thing we know of to keep our brains healthy and reduce the risk of cognitive decline. We'll discuss this topic in more detail in Chapter 5.

The second type of activity referenced by the C.A.P.E. model is *social activity*. More attention has been paid to this area lately as scientists have considered the positive impact of social engagement on emotional health and the detrimental effects of social isolation. We also see that from a cognitive standpoint, regularly interacting with friends, family members, or coworkers is associated with better brain skills.

While you might not think intuitively that spending time with a friend is exercising your brain, consider the complexities of social encounters (particularly good ones). As you attend and listen to your friend, you're considering his or her thoughts, perspectives, and feelings, and then you use this information to provide a thoughtful response, perhaps sharing your own experiences in the process. Social interaction is both a remarkable human accomplishment *and* something that requires considerable brain horsepower. The many cognitive abilities used during even simple conversations— paying attention to what the person is expressing verbally and nonverbally, mentally juggling the details of the conversation (an example of *working memory*), trying to consider the person's perspective (what's called *theory of mind*)—certainly give the brain a thorough workout. We'll consider how social engagement impacts the brain in Chapter 6.

The third part of the "A" in the C.A.P.E. model (and the last part of what I like to call the "activity triad") is *mental or intellectual activity*. Mental activity takes many forms; a few include reading, doing crossword puzzles, playing musical instruments, and going to museums. Staying mentally active at school or work certainly counts, as does managing a busy household with multiple schedules and events to keep track of. Mental activity remains important throughout life, and stretching the brain by learning new things or pushing ourselves intellectually pays significant neurological dividends.

The science indicates that people who are more involved in mental activities tend to show fewer cognitive changes (particularly decline) in midlife and beyond and are at less risk of developing dementia. There are some really interesting studies looking at large groups of people who are and are not mentally active, and the results are often quite striking in terms of how the brains of both groups are working. We'll come back to this topic in Chapter 7.

Incidentally, activities that include multiple aspects of the activity triad can be particularly powerful for the brain; think playing tennis or racquetball, which have strong physical and social components, or volunteer work, which can be mentally stimulating and often involves lots of social activity.

Moving on, the next part of the C.A.P.E. model, the "P," refers to *prevention of cognitive problems*. We now know of many factors that contribute to diminished brain health. By modifying these factors, we may be able to improve how our brain works and possibly even prevent some types of dementia.

For example, there is evidence that diets with lots of saturated fat are bad for the heart—and the brain too. In contrast, people who adhere to a Mediterranean-style diet seem to have brains that are more efficient at processing information and remembering new things. This type of diet includes lots of fruits and vegetables, olive oil, certain types of nuts (like walnuts), beans, fish, and a little wine, with little to no red meat or dairy products. We'll look at the science of nutrition and the brain in detail in Chapter 8.

We also know that managing stress effectively is another way to prevent problems with attention, memory, and other thinking skills. Reducing stress protects certain brain structures (such as the hippocampus, a vital memory region) from being bathed in potentially toxic hormones that are released when we feel chronically tense. Sleep difficulties, some medical problems, and smoking can really reduce brain horsepower too. In Chapters 9 to 11, we'll talk more about these and other factors we can manage to potentially prevent cognitive problems.

The final part of the C.A.P.E. model is the "E," which stands for *education about the brain*. The entire book essentially covers this part of the model, although Chapter 12 has a particular focus on strategies to lock in new brain-boosting habits based on our understanding of how the brain works.

The myths noted earlier represent just a fraction of misguided beliefs that many people hold about the brain and our thinking skills, often through no fault of their own. As a neuropsychologist, I often see patients who are concerned that they are having "memory problems," when in fact they are experiencing increased stress, anxiety, or depression that leads them to perceive that their memory isn't what it used to be. Some of my work, in turn, involves helping people understand that appropriate stress management or treatment of emotional concerns can lead to better perceptions of how their memory is working.

In a related vein, when people feel that their memory is failing them, they may be noticing normal age-related changes to their thinking skills. While frustrating and embarrassing at times, these changes do not necessarily portend serious cognitive disorders such as dementia. We actually begin to experience some reduction in our processing speed and name retrieval when we're in our forties. Our life experience and wisdom help us compensate for these lapses, but they can certainly be annoying. Having realistic expectations for what our brain does well and where it may slip up from time to time can be reassuring.

Now that I've laid out many of the topics we'll be covering in this book, I wanted to offer an opportunity to consider the types of brain-promoting activities you currently engage in. Take a quick look at the following, which are questions from a measure I developed with some colleagues called the Cognitive Health Questionnaire, and rate yourself:

1. How much light physical activity or exercise do you get in a typical week? (Note: One period of activity is 20 to

30+ minutes of mild exercise from gardening, general housework, bicycle repair, slow walking, and so on.)

_____ None or minimal (0 points)

_____ One period of activity (1 point)

_____ Two periods of activity (2 points)

_____ Three periods of activity (3 points)

_____ More than three periods of activity (4 points)

2. How much moderate or vigorous physical activity or exercise do you get in a typical week? (Note: One workout is 20 to 30+ minutes of moderate exercise from brisk walking, hiking, jogging, cycling, swimming, working out at the gym, dancing, and so on.)

_____ None or minimal (0 points)

_____ One workout (1 point)

_____ Two workouts (2 points)

_____ Three workouts (3 points)

_____ More than three workouts (4 points)

3. How often do you socialize with family members other than your partner in a typical week? (Note: Socializing = interacting with someone other than your partner for at least 10 minutes at a time.)

_____ Never or rarely (0 points)

_____ Once (1 point)

_____ Twice (2 points)

_____ Three times (3 points)

_____ More than three times (4 points)

4. How often do you socialize with friends in a typical week? (Note: Socializing = interacting with someone other than your partner for at least 10 minutes at a time.)

_____ Never or rarely (0 points)

_____ Once (1 point)

_____ Twice (2 points)

_____ Three times (3 points)

_____ More than three times (4 points)

5. How many times per week do you do something that makes you consider or remember new information? (Note: Activities might include reading a newspaper, magazine, or book for at least 10 minutes; going to a museum or art gallery; doing crossword puzzles or Sudoku.)

_____ Never or rarely (0 points)

_____ Once (1 point)

_____ Twice (2 points)

_____ Three times (3 points)

_____ More than three times (4 points)

6. How many times in a typical week do you use strategies or techniques to help you remember or organize information? (Note: Strategies might include using a paper or computer calendar; writing lists or notes; using mental images of things you need to remember; using an alarm clock or smartphone alarms.)

_____ Never or rarely (0 points)

_____ Once (1 point)

_____ Twice (2 points)

_____ Three times (3 points)

_____ More than three times (4 points)

Now, for questions 1 to 6, tally your responses. Here's a general interpretation you can use for your total score:

0 to 6: You're not doing much in terms of activities that could help your brain. You might want to read most if not all of this book to get some ideas on how to add activities into your daily routine.

7 to 14: You engage in some brain-healthy activities but could probably ramp up your efforts. You may want to read specific chapters related to areas where you're not doing too much right now.

15+: You're doing a lot of the right things to maintain if not improve how your brain is working. This book can help supplement what you're already doing and potentially give you new ideas to scale up your efforts even further.

Also, try this one:

How many of the following strategies do you use in a typical week to help you remember or organize information? (Check all that apply.)

_____ Paper organizer/calendar/planner (such as an
        appointment book)
_____ Computer or smartphone organizer/calendar
_____ Wall calendar
_____ Sticky notes or other notes
_____ Lists (e.g., grocery lists, daily to-do lists, checklists)
_____ Kitchen timers or smartphone alarms
_____ Creating mental images of things you need to
        remember
_____ Grouping or "clustering" new information together
        (e.g., using an acronym such as CLOG to remember
        to go to the *cleaners, library, office,* and *grocery store*)
_____ Putting new information in rhymes or stories

For this last item, you should probably be using a minimum
of two to three strategies listed above (or two to three related
strategies that might not be listed here). This question relates
to content in Chapter 4, so if you're looking to boost your
strategy use, you might start there.

We've got many interesting brain health topics to delve
into, so let's get to it. I hope you'll enjoy and be stimulated by the material in the chapters to come. Perhaps more
important, my goal is to introduce concepts that you can
begin applying to your life immediately to put you on the
road to building a better brain.

How Does Neuroscience Relate to Brain Health?

NEUROSCIENCE IS EVERYWHERE. WHILE YOU MAY not always recognize it as such, articles in newspapers and magazines, online pieces, morning talk shows, and evening news programs regularly cover the brain. In a community course I teach on promoting brain health, we start class with a "media roundup," where students bring in articles they've found in popular culture so we can discuss them. It never ceases to amaze me how widespread material about the brain is nowadays.

While the amount of media coverage related to neuroscience is generally very positive, it is also important to note that brain research can be misused and misinterpreted. Distilling complex research findings into, for example, a short blurb in a newspaper column or a sound bite on network news usually obscures the nitty-gritty details of the study. In this chapter, we'll discuss some neuroscience basics to give

you an introduction to related concepts. My hope is that this information will come in handy while reading this book and as you wade through content in the popular media.

NEUROSCIENCE PRIMER

Let's start with a few general facts about the brain. It weighs about 3 pounds, which is remarkably light considering the vast computing, processing, and reasoning powers it contains. Central to its powers are brain cells, or neurons (Figure 2.1)—about 100 billion of them. Each neuron is linked with many other neurons, totaling about 1 trillion connections. Just for perspective, consider that there are 400 billion stars in the Milky Way Galaxy—fewer than half of the connections within the human brain! All of these connections allow us to engage in myriad activities and experiences in daily life: talking, listening, remembering, walking, feeling, reflecting, attending, and so on.

Our neurons are also unique compared to other cells in the body in that they communicate with each other and are capable of significant growth and restructuring.

Regarding the latter, as seen in Figure 2.1, the cell body of the neuron has branches extending from it, referred to as *dendrites* (derived from the Greek word for "tree"). The dendrites are responsible for critically important brain tasks, such as gathering information from other neurons to help improve the "conversations" neurons have with one another. They also grow and adapt throughout our entire

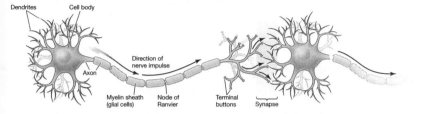

FIGURE 2.1 Structures of a Neuron

Source: Figure 3.5 in Psychological Science, fifth edition, by Michael Gazzaniga, Todd Heatherton, and Diane Halpern. Copyright © 2016, 2013, 2010, 2006, 2003 by W.W. Norton & Company, Inc. Used by permission of W.W. Norton & Company, Inc.

life span. Some activities, including intellectual enrichment, are known to sprout new dendrites, presumably leading to more cross talk between neurons throughout the brain.

The brain also contains a wide variety of specialized chemicals—neurotransmitters—that help messages travel from one neuron to another. You may have heard of some neurotransmitters (let's call them "NTs"), particularly as they relate to certain behaviors, feelings, or medications. One example is serotonin, which is an essential NT for regulating our mood. Serotonin is targeted by certain antidepressant medications such as Prozac and Zoloft, which serve to boost serotonin levels and reduce depression and anxiety.

Another commonly studied NT is norepinephrine, which plays an important role in attention, arousal, and motivation. Some attention-deficit/hyperactivity disorder

(ADHD) medications increase norepinephrine levels, leading to better ability to focus. Dopamine is often considered to be the "pleasure" NT, which gets released when we're engaging in stimulating or pleasurable activities, like eating a great meal, having sex, or skiing. It's also involved in regulating physical movement, and it breaks down in some conditions like Parkinson's disease.

While it's tempting to view NTs somewhat simplistically, they are anything but. Changes in one NT impact not only other NTs but the chemical regulation of the brain itself. It's also known that certain activities, particularly exercise, can increase NT levels (and do a variety of other positive things to the brain).

Neurons are always working hard, so they need and deserve their own support staff. This is where neurotrophins come into play. Neurotrophins help to build and maintain neurons, increase NT levels, and improve the way blood flows throughout the brain. One commonly studied neurotrophin is called brain-derived neurotrophic factor, or BDNF. BDNF has been referred to as the "Miracle-Gro" of the brain given its powerful and nurturing effects on neurons. One of the benefits of exercise is its tendency to increase the amount of BDNF available to support the brain's billions of neurons; we'll discuss this in more detail later in the book.

In terms of brain structures, we could devote an entire book to the topic of neuroanatomy, but you're probably not reading this book for that reason. Let me just highlight a few regions that will be particularly relevant for us here. The brain's outer layer is called the *cerebral cortex* (*cortex* being a Latin term for "tree bark"). The cortex is divided into four subdivisions or lobes, which can be remembered by the acronym FPOT: frontal, parietal, occipital, and temporal.

Take a look at Figure 2.2 to get a sense of what the cerebral cortex looks like. Note that as with other brain structures, we can describe each lobe of the cortex in the singular (like the "frontal lobe"); we can also use the plural ("frontal lobes"), particularly if we're referencing the left and right sides of the lobe. Another option to describe cortical regions is to use terms like "frontal cortex" or "temporal cortex."

The frontal lobes play a critical role in many uniquely human abilities and can even grow in response to some life-

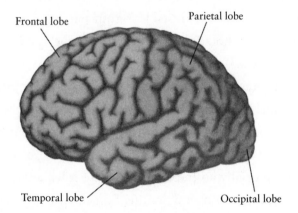

FIGURE 2.2 The Four Lobes of the Cerebral Cortex

Source: *Figure 4.1 in* The Neuroscience of Psychotherapy: Building and Rebuilding the Human Brain *by Louis Cozolino. Copyright © 2002 by Louis J. Cozolino. Used by permission of W.W. Norton & Company, Inc.*

style activities (including exercise). Most neuroscientists also believe that the frontal lobes are the home of our executive functions. We'll discuss executive functions more in the next chapter, but in short, these are cognitive skills that help us engage in goal-directed behaviors. So, if we need to get started on a new task (like cleaning the garage), we need to plan and organize our approach (start in the back of the garage and move forward), persist through the task (decide what to throw away and what to keep), stay flexible in our approach (take a break when we're hungry or thirsty, or when a neighbor stops by to see if he or she can get a good deal on some tools we've decided to sell), and ultimately complete what we're trying to do (have a garage sale and make a few bucks).

There are also a variety of regions underneath the cerebral cortex, which are referred to as *subcortical* regions. One that is particularly notable for our purposes is the hippocampus, a seahorse-shaped structure in the middle of the brain (Figure 2.3).

Simply put, the hippocampus is more important for what most people think of as "memory" than any other structure in the brain. Research beginning many years ago found that damage to the hippocampus inevitably results in memory deficits, especially an impaired ability to learn and remember new information in daily life. Someone who helped us learn a great deal about the hippocampus—and the negative effects of damage there—was known by most neuroscientists only by his initials: H.M.

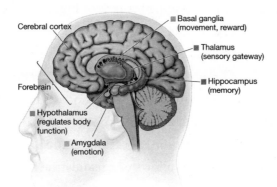

FIGURE 2.3 Subcortical Regions of the Brain

Source: Figure 3.24 in Psychological Science, *fifth edition, by Michael Gazzaniga, Todd Heatherton, and Diane Halpern. Copyright © 2016, 2013, 2010, 2006, 2003 by W.W. Norton & Company, Inc. Used by permission of W.W. Norton & Company, Inc.*

H.M. had intractable epilepsy, and his neurosurgeon believed that removing most of his hippocampus (an area of the brain where seizures can originate) would reduce or eliminate his seizures. The subsequent surgery was a success. H.M. no longer had seizures. However, despite this life-altering change, he would never be able to live independently again. Why? From that day forward, he was essentially unable to remember anything new—the names of his doctors, recent news, even what he had for breakfast an hour earlier. As the title of a recent book on H.M. noted, he was stuck in "Permanent Present Tense." His dramatic example helped neuroscientists understand the importance of the hippocampus for learning and remembering new informa-

tion, primarily by studying his lack of both after his conse-
quential surgery.

With modern brain science, we no longer need to rely on
case studies of brain damage to learn how the brain works (or
doesn't). In fact, we can now consider not just brain dysfunction and pathology but also the opposite: *the process of brain
growth and development* throughout the entire life span. State-
of-the-art neuroscience allows us to study the healthy brain,
rather than focus exclusively on the diseased or injured one.

The hippocampus was and continues to be a shining
star of this research. As we'll discuss later in the book,
early research looking at the effects of exercise on the brain
found that the hippocampus responds powerfully to exercise. Unlike what was considered neurological dogma until
fairly recently, we in fact grow new neurons in the hippocampus when we exercise, and these neurons are associated with improved ability to learn and remember. More
recent studies have continued to reinforce the connection
between physical fitness and growth in the hippocampus.

GENETICS AND NEUROSCIENCE

The area of genetics, as related to neuroscience, is very "hot"
right now. We are learning about genes that are involved
in different cognitive skills, such as memory and executive
functioning, as well as genes that may increase our risk for
Alzheimer's disease. One genetic factor, in particular, is
called *APOE-ε4*, which refers to the ε4 allele of the apolipo-

protein E gene. For some time now, we've known that this gene is a risk factor for developing dementia. In other words, if you take a specialized test for this gene and it comes up positive, you are more likely than the average person in the general population to develop Alzheimer's. While this is certainly a scary proposition, it's also important to note that your risk increases *somewhat* with this gene, and it by no means indicates that you *will* get dementia in the future.

A more optimistic take on *APOE-ε4* has recently emerged. While we know that this is a risk factor for cognitive problems, there is also evidence that if you have this gene, you are more likely to derive brain-related benefits from some lifestyle activities—particularly exercise—than the average person. This may seem counterintuitive based on the Alzheimer's research I mentioned above, although *APOE-ε4* is increasingly considered to be a *plasticity* gene. Plasticity refers to the ability of the brain to change and respond to the environment. We'll discuss plasticity in more detail later in the chapter, but for now, keep in mind that some genes appear to do double duty, carrying both aspects of risk and potential benefit for the brain.

BRAIN-RELATED CHANGES IN ADULTHOOD

We've all had what are called *cognitive lapses*. That is, the experience of forgetting why we entered a room down the hall, where we were going mid-conversation, or what the name of that darn thingy is over there. Most people have had minor problems finding their car in the parking lot at a mall or after grocery shopping. These experiences are fairly common, and—though frustrating and maybe embarrassing—totally normal. Our brains are prone to these mild lapses, and at some level they are part of being human. The stereotype of the "absent-minded professor" actually applies to all of us at some point, and that's okay.

It's important not to pathologize these little slips we experience. Sometimes people come to see a neuropsychologist like myself when they notice an increase in these lapses, but the ramp up in frequency does not necessarily herald a cognitive disorder. As we'll discuss throughout the book, particularly in Chapter 3, cognitive lapses come from many sources. Fortunately, many of them do not represent dementia or other forms of cognitive impairment.

That being said, there are cognitive changes that are more troubling. Leaving one's keys in the dishwasher, repeatedly asking the same question every few minutes, or forgetting how to use common appliances all warrant more concern than typical lapses in memory. Mismanaging one's finances or medications would also fall into this category. Along these lines, I wanted to mention a few types of cognitive disorders that can occur in adulthood, particularly as we get into our sixties and beyond.

The first is what's called *mild cognitive impairment*, or *MCI*. MCI is a diagnostic category that is used when someone is still functioning pretty well in daily life—that is, manages medications, pays bills, cooks, and drives without significant difficulties—but nevertheless reports having memory problems and shows memory or other deficits on cognitive tests. MCI is a double-edged sword of sorts; on the one hand, those with MCI are at increased risk for developing dementia in the future (particularly Alzheimer's disease). In fact, every year, approximately 10% of people with MCI "convert" to dementia.

On the other hand, some people with MCI remain stable cognitively and do not move into the dementia category. We don't know as much about those who have a more stable MCI course, or those who were initially diagnosed with MCI and show improvement rather than decline. However, regardless of the direction MCI may go, being in the MCI category is an opportunity for intervention. Using more memory and organizational strategies, increasing physical and social activity, and making good dietary and other lifestyle choices may help some of us stay cognitively healthy, even if we have slipped a bit.

In this context, I'd like to point your attention to an image that helps clarify different possible cognitive "trajectories" (Figure 2.4).

I find this image elegant and informative, particularly because I see these trajectories play out in my clinic. Just to orient you, these four hypothetical cognitive paths through life essentially reflect the good (A), the bad (D), the average (B), and the reformed (C). Note that the line indicating the *functional threshold* is the point at which someone needs help from others to manage his or her daily activities.

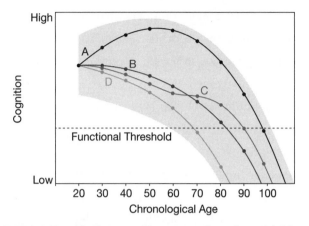

FIGURE 2.4 Possible Cognitive Trajectories throughout Adulthood

Source: Reproduced with permission of Sage Publications, Journals, via Copyright Clearance Center, Inc.; from "Enrichment Effects on Adult Cognitive Development," Christopher Hertzog et al. (2009), Psychological Science in the Public Interest, 9, p. 8.

First off, we can think of a person falling on the A trajectory as a brain health superstar: someone who has sought out enriching experiences throughout life, made good decisions related to diet and sleep, and stayed physically and socially active. The figure proposes that this person may not need any assistance with daily functioning related to bill payment, cooking, or medication management until she is in late life. Certainly something to strive for. B reflects more of a typical trajectory; the average adult who makes some good wellness-oriented decisions and choices, exercises at times but perhaps not consistently, and uses a few organizational strategies such as an appointment book or lists.

C is the path that some of my patients seem to be on. If you look at the trajectory of this one, you can see that around age 60, the individual has decided to make some changes that improve his brain health in a noticeable way. Maybe he's been diagnosed with MCI and feels that he needs to start exercising more or join a book club to become more mentally and socially engaged. As a function of these types of changes, he bumps out his cognitive health trajectory in such a way that he has a lower risk of further cognitive changes. I have seen a fair amount of people in this category, and it's inspiring to observe their shifts in perspective after getting a wake-up call of sorts.

Finally, the D path is what I think of as a "cognitive couch potato." That is, someone who has tended not to take care of himself or herself well throughout life (for a wide variety of possible reasons) and subsequently experiences cognitive decline much faster than others. While there are some factors out of our control (such as genetics) that are not represented in this figure, this book is dedicated to clarifying the things we know we can do in daily life that can potentially help us stay out of the D trajectory.

Coming back to our discussion of cognitive disorders, note that dementia is a frequently misunderstood diagnostic category. Dementia is a broad umbrella term that includes a variety of separate diseases or conditions. Alzheimer's disease is one form of dementia, but there are many others. These include frontotemporal dementia, Lewy body dementia, or vascular dementia. While the types of cognitive problems associated with each condition can differ, there are a few common features in dementia. Fundamentally, dementia is characterized by problems with multiple cognitive skills and a breakdown in one's ability to complete daily tasks adequately and independently. While memory impairment is the hallmark feature of dementia, problems with executive functioning skills (including organization, planning, and initiating and completing tasks), language, attention, and spatial abilities can also occur.

The time course of dementia varies from person to person. The early stages include cognitive problems and functional decline, and later stages involve incapacity and the need for consistent care from others. As we'll discuss in later chapters, the bleak outlook of one's dementia course can be tempered somewhat by engaging in brain-boosting activities, such as exercise and mental stimulation. These types of activities allow some people to decline less rapidly than might have been the case otherwise. So, even in the case of dementia, it remains possible to exert some control over the disease process.

PLASTICITY AND COGNITIVE RESERVE

One of the most important concepts in modern neuroscience is that of *plasticity*, or, more specifically, *neuroplasticity*. This concept relates to the brain's ability to adapt to new experiences. Years ago, it was believed that the brain was set in stone after adolescence, and that the only direction it could go was down. Medical professionals were under the impression that people simply became more forgetful, more distracted, and less organized with age. While we could learn to manage these changes, it was believed that there really wasn't much we could do to improve how the brain worked.

We now know that the brain's development is dynamic: it changes throughout life in many ways. **Of particular importance for our purposes here, lifestyle choices are known to shape the brain and cognitive skills positively.** In a sense, much of this book is based around the idea of plasticity: we have the ability to proactively rewire our brains if we adopt positive habits, live in certain ways, and engage in novel and stimulating activities. Conversely, making less ideal decisions about our lifestyles can have negative effects on how the brain operates.

One fascinating example of research that relates to brain plasticity was conducted with taxi drivers in London. These drivers have a dizzying array of streets to memorize and navigate in their line of work. This was a particularly compelling group to study, given the spatial memory demands required as a taxi driver, and researchers used structural neuroimaging to determine whether their brains differed from similarly aged people who didn't drive taxis. The scientists paid particular attention to the hippocampus, the brain structure we discussed earlier that plays a critical role in learning and retrieving information.

Study results indicated that the cabbies' brains were indeed different. Their hippocampus—on both sides of the brain—was larger than that of other people. Even more interesting was the finding that the longer someone had been a taxi driver, the larger a region of their right hippocampus was; note that the right side of the hippocampus is linked to spatial memory. In other words, engaging in a certain activity consistently over time had a direct influence on brain development. This is just one of a number of studies demonstrating how responsive the brain is to new experiences, a theme we'll come back to as we discuss different ways to improve brain health.

A related concept is *cognitive reserve*. Cognitive reserve refers to how certain life experiences have a protective effect on how the brain works and ages. Some life experiences— such as how much education you have attained, how stimulating your job is, and your general intellectual ability—are particularly important factors. In fact, people with more education under their belts and who have mentally demanding jobs (including managing others) are less likely to develop dementia. Even if dementia does occur, it may emerge at a more advanced age than in those with less cognitive reserve. So, this concept explains some of the differences between people's cognitive skills, and mental decline, later in life.

We should also distinguish between *passive* cognitive reserve and *active* reserve. For many years, the research in this area related mostly to a few key types of passive reserve: how many years of education you have completed, and how intellectually gifted you are. While these factors are certainly important, a more recent twist on reserve relates to what someone might be doing *throughout* life on an active and ongoing basis. Active reserve is something that we can continually build that adds to our brain's ability to function at its highest level.

Take mental stimulation as one example. Going through college is a very mentally (and socially) stimulating process, and certainly shapes our brain to think and reason in new ways. But what about after college? And what about people who haven't been to college or never finished? There is increasing evidence that staying mentally stimulated through reading, taking community courses, playing a musical instrument, or engaging in other brain-stretching activities helps promote new brain growth and supplements our cognitive reserve.

Some research has examined how life experiences, education, and other factors buffer the effects of brain-related disease. In an early study, over 600 nuns agreed to undergo cognitive testing every few years, and they also graciously agreed to donate their brains to the researchers upon death. Quite a gift, to be sure. The findings were remarkable at the time and continue to be so: despite having essentially intact cognitive skills during life and functioning at a high level up until their demise, the brains of many of these nuns had neurofibrillary tangles and other pathological findings identical to what is observed in Alzheimer's disease. In other words, their brains looked like they were from individuals with a common form of dementia, even though the nuns didn't actually show symptoms of dementia while living.

Another intriguing finding from the so-called Nun

Study: complex ideas expressed in nuns' early-adulthood writing samples—an indicator of intellectual ability and passive cognitive reserve—were associated with a decreased chance of developing dementia. This observation was highly novel and supported the idea that early life experiences have significant implications for our brain health many years down the road. It's also likely that the nuns' social and mental engagement throughout their lives (active cognitive reserve) played a critical role in their ability to withstand the effects of a devastating brain disease.

Another study conducted more recently studied a group of older adults, some of whom eventually developed dementia. The researchers were particularly interested in one lifestyle factor that is known to have positive effects on the brain and our thinking skills: social activity. During the study, people were given tests to measure their cognitive abilities, and they were asked questions about their social ties. Then, after their demise, their brains were examined in detail.

The results supported the importance of active cognitive reserve from a social standpoint: those with the richest social networks were much more effective at maintaining their memory and language skills over time, even when their brains showed signs of dementia. In other words, having many connections with others seemed to reduce the impact of negative brain changes on important thinking skills.

These and other studies collectively demonstrate that

certain types of activity we engage in—activities that build our cognitive reserve—have rejuvenating effects on the brain. We'll consider the implications of related research throughout the book, particularly regarding areas such as mental activity, social engagement, and exercise.

The Cognitive Trio That Matters Most: Attention, Memory, and Executive Functions

RON WAS REFERRED TO ME AFTER MENTIONING TO his primary-care physician, and then to his neurologist, that he was becoming increasingly forgetful. He was still doing relatively well in his work as a computer programmer, but he was having more trouble remembering details from recent conversations, focusing on tasks, and retrieving names of people he knew relatively well. A magnetic resonance imaging (MRI) scan of his brain had not revealed anything out of the ordinary, and he didn't have a history of medical problems that could account for his reported cognitive decline.

My evaluation with Ron was mostly unremarkable from a cognitive standpoint—his memory and other thinking skills were essentially normal across a large battery of neuropsychological tests—but it was more than apparent that he had been under considerable stress and was showing signs of depression. I concluded that he did not have a cognitive disorder, and that his stress and depression were making him feel inattentive and amnesic. I surmised that managing his stress more effectively and treating his depression would potentially improve his quality of life and his cognitive health. I saw him about a year later, and after switching jobs and getting counseling to help improve his mood, his perceived memory problems had mostly remitted. It was reassuring to observe that his cognitive lapses were in fact reversible; with the right treatment and a better job, he saw a clear uptick in his thinking skills in daily life.

Ron's case brings up a few issues: How do we describe our thinking skills? What do our beliefs about our abilities represent? Do our cognitive concerns relate to measurable cognitive impairment or to other factors, such as stress? As we'll see, how we talk about our own cognitive abilities is sometimes at odds with what's actually happening (or not happening) within our brains. There also are three key aspects of brain functioning that figure more heavily into our daily lives than others, and we'll discuss this "cognitive trio" later in the chapter.

HOW ACCURATELY DO WE DESCRIBE OUR COGNITIVE SKILLS?

People in the general population often have cognitive lapses—it's part of being human. In fact, about half of people report memory problems, and at least a third say that they have trouble finding the right word to use in conversation, forget where they park the car, and misplace their car keys. We shouldn't view these experiences as representing memory failures. On the contrary, minor episodes of forgetfulness are merely evidence that we're just like everyone else.

More generally, when we experience memory lapses or problems concentrating, what are we actually noticing? Believe it or not, our so-called *cognitive complaints* relate to a number of different experiences and observations. First, we could be detecting age-related cognitive changes that, while annoying and potentially distressing, are entirely normal. Another possibility is that we're noticing actual cognitive changes that are detectable on sensitive neuropsychological tests. In other words, if I were to notice that I was increasingly forgetful in daily life, there's a possibility that cognitive measures would indicate that I was having true memory or other problems. However, it's important to note that our reported cognitive lapses are only mildly linked to actual performance on objective cognitive tests, so neuropsychologists such as myself need to consider other factors too.

An additional source for memory complaints is our mood state. Depression, in particular, tends to color our daily experience so globally that just about anything we describe about ourselves tends to be negative, including our perceptions of how our brain is working. Many studies have found that people who report problems with cognitive skills tend to be depressed, anxious, or under some form of stress or tension. Like stressed-out Ron, we might be picking up on something mood-related that makes us feel like we're slipping cognitively but is actually unrelated to a brain disorder per se. Medical symptoms such as chronic pain can also be stressful and lead us to feel inattentive or forgetful.

It's interesting to note that concerns about one cognitive skill may actually reflect problems with another one. A study some colleagues and I did a few years ago revealed that memory complaints relate to cognitive abilities other than memory—for example, with processing speed, or how quickly and efficiently we process information. So, when we feel that our memory is slipping, we might actually be noticing a change in another brain-related ability.

Some research has also found that the way we describe our cognitive skills depends on how physically active we are. One study with older adults found that people who were more physically fit reported fewer instances of forgetting in daily life (and also had more brain volume in the memory-critical hippocampus). It seems that if we're exercising a fair amount day to day, we tend to notice fewer cognitive problems than if we're more sedentary. This also makes sense in the context of the many brain-related benefits we experience from physical activity, which we'll take a deep dive into in Chapter 5.

Another perspective is from Daniel Kahneman, the Nobel Prize–winning psychologist who has researched many fresh and novel ideas about how the brain works in daily life. One of his ideas, backed up by considerable research, is what he calls the "peak-end rule." When recalling a past experience, the peak-end rule states that we tend to overvalue the most painful "peak" of an experience and the end of the experience compared to the rest of the experience.

This rule can be applied to reports of cognitive problems. Over the years, some folks I've met with in my clinic have cited a few isolated but salient and troubling memory lapses they've had: forgetting to pick up their child after ballet practice, missing the due date on a phone bill resulting in a threated service termination, or running into a former coworker in the grocery store and forgetting their name. These are often distressing experiences and stick with us as apparent reminders of our declining cognitive skills.

However, and along the lines of the peak-end rule, we tend to discount the many day-to-day experiences we have when we *don't* forget things, because these aren't cause for concern and usually aren't very noticeable (for example, paying the bills on time for 6 months straight; attending nearly all medical appointments that have been scheduled). In fact, it might be useful to take a step back and consider whether the episode of forgetfulness that concerns us represents a pattern we've been noticing or something more isolated.

Descriptions of cognitive problems can also vary based on who we associate with the most, and on how old we are. Kids and adolescents are around others with learning and attention challenges, so they tend to describe problems with "focus" and being disorganized, perhaps for this reason. Middle-aged and older adults are more likely to report problems with memory, because this is often what they see others struggling with in their age group.

One of the most common cognitive complaints relates to having problems finding the right words to use in conversation, referred to as *word-finding difficulties*. This issue usually crops up in our forties and worsens some—usually mildly—from there on out. While some people report long-standing problems remembering names, increased difficulties with this skill are usually related to normal and subtle breakdowns in the connections between parts of the brain that store "name" information and "face" information.

Curiously, very few people report having problems with facial recognition—if you've seen someone at least a few times, you'll probably recognize them again—which makes sense from an evolutionary standpoint. Thousands of years ago, it didn't really matter what someone was called, or whether a fellow hunter-gatherer even had a rudimentary name. More important was the ability to recognize whether this person was aggressive, kind, generous, or indifferent. Fast forward to the present day, where despite our ability to describe many aspects of our environment, we tend to forget names of people and objects as we age. The brain is simply wired to remember some things better than others.

COGNITIVE TRIO PART 1: ATTENTION

In the last section, we discussed how we describe our cognitive skills, but note that the examples I used primarily related to memory. Unless you've studied cognition and the brain, you may not be familiar with the rich smorgasbord of

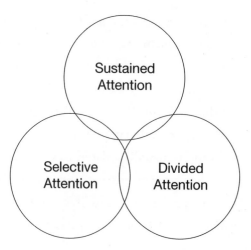

FIGURE 3.1 Types of Attention

cognitive functions generated by the brain—there's a whole lot more than just memory. We'll start our discussion of the "cognitive trio" with attention and its various "flavors," then describe multiple aspects of memory and the brain's executive functions.

Attention is a multifaceted concept: it has three key skills that are unique but overlap somewhat (Figure 3.1).

The first key attentional skill is *sustained attention*: our ability to focus for an extended period of time. In some ways, this is the foundation for anything we do in daily life. In order to learn and absorb new material (like someone's name or details from a conversation), we have to be able to sit still, attend, and listen. If our boss has something important to say (at least from his or her perspective), we need to be able to "pay attention" to what's being said. If we're taking a class or attending a seminar, it's imperative that we keep our focus for a while and not daydream or become distracted.

Next is *selective attention*. This ability helps us focus on one thing while ignoring something else. When you're in a conversation in a busy restaurant, are you able to tune out the background noise—other diners, dishes breaking in the kitchen, the ambient music you're not crazy about? The brain is usually fairly effective at ignoring extraneous information that we would otherwise see or hear, particularly when our experience in the moment is interesting and engrossing. Incidentally, selective attention, as with sustained attention, is often reduced in individuals with ADHD (more on this condition later).

Another attentional skill is *divided attention*. This is the fancy term for the more commonly used one, *multitasking*. Divided attention essentially refers to how well we can switch from one task to another and distribute our focus across more than one thing at a time. There are both benefits and risks to dividing our attention in this way. On the positive side, if we have practiced a skill repeatedly—at a level where we're not even thinking about it—adding something else to the mix may go relatively well.

Consider the example of driving a car. When learning to drive, you had to divide your attention across multiple subtasks, including handling the wheel, putting the right amount of pressure on the accelerator or the brake, using the turn signal, and so on, all while focusing on the road ahead, the driver behind you, and any cars or pedestrians off to either side. Talk about information overload. Over time, though, managing the physical and cognitive aspects of driving became easier, and eventually you stopped thinking about all the details. Your brain had developed a *motor program* that involved dividing attention in ways you were (and are) consciously unaware of.

On a more concerning note, dividing attention across tasks that are relatively new, effortful, and detail-oriented is fraught with peril. The brain is simply better designed to "unitask" than to "multitask." A seminal study conducted a few years ago proved this point with a fair dose of irony. People were asked to indicate how often they typically multitasked with media—things like watching online videos or TV, Web surfing, listening to music, composing e-mails—and self-reported low and high multitasking groups were then compared on cognitive tasks that assessed various skills. The findings revealed that those who claimed to multitask the most, and felt that they were good at it, performed *worse* on actual tests of multitasking. Put another way, people were better at managing multiple things during the study if they described themselves as being less scattered in daily life. So, the next time someone you know says, "I'm a great multitasker," look at him askance with a sly, knowing grin, and emphasize that he might want to rethink his perspective.

Importantly, when people report having "memory" problems, the real problem might actually be with attention. If we don't focus well on what we hear or see, it's simply harder to remember it. As we discussed earlier, stress can certainly affect our ability to concentrate, so people under stress tend to report having more problems in this regard, even though their cognitive challenges are temporary (and will likely remit once they've managed their stress effectively or the stressful circumstance passes).

Some people have a diagnosable attentional disorder, otherwise known as ADHD. This is a developmental condition that interferes with some aspects of functioning at school, home, and maybe elsewhere, usually in childhood but sometimes not until adolescence. In those who are very bright or who have lots of support (such as parents or tutors who provide considerable structure and guidance with homework, studying, and the like), the symptoms of ADHD may not have as much of an impact on daily life. My experience is that some of these people show the most struggles in college, when the structure they've been accustomed to throughout their development is suddenly removed and they're left to fend for themselves. But note that there is no such thing as adult-*onset* ADHD, only ADHD that may not have been formally diagnosed earlier in life but was always present at some level.

COGNITIVE TRIO PART 2: MEMORY

Karen was in her mid-sixties and noticed increasing problems with her memory. She emphasized that there were some things she remembered well and other things that faded pretty quickly. As she said, "I can tell you all about my career, good times I had in high school and college, even details from soccer games from when I was a kid. My friends still tell me that I've got a good working vocabulary. It's the stuff that happened yesterday that I'm having trouble drawing up." Cognitive testing revealed difficulties learning new material that I asked her to remember—such as learning and later recalling a long list of words—but no detectable problems in other areas. In fact, her ability to remember information from long ago remained strong, and she was also effective at repeating brief bits of material, such as short sequences of random numbers.

Memory can be divided up in a number of ways, although what we often notice slipping in midlife and beyond—as Karen did—is what's called *episodic memory*. This form of memory refers to our memory for certain events (or episodes) and related details that we experience day to day. Content from a conversation we recently had with a friend, the time we tried that new restaurant, and what we had for breakfast all count.

Research on memory often looks specifically at episodic memory, which is usually measured by how well someone can learn and later recall a list of words, a story, or visual information like faces or designs. This is also an important area measured by clinical neuropsychologists and other brain-oriented professionals. Episodic memory tends to show mild age-related decline over the years but can also be enhanced by exercise, being socially active, and taking on mentally stimulating hobbies. Suffice it to say that episodic memory can be improved or left to wilt on the vine depending in part on lifestyle choices we make. We'll be talking much more about related brain-enriching activities in the chapters ahead.

Semantic memory refers to what Karen mentioned without concern—memory for words, facts, and other general knowledge we've picked up over the years. This type of memory is relatively resistant to change, even in the face of brain injury and mild forms of dementia. We can certainly struggle to draw up the right word in conversation—the age-related word-finding difficulties we considered earlier—but we usually can retrieve the word given some time.

Have you ever walked into a room at home and forgotten why you went there? Or been told someone's name and mentally misplaced it a few seconds later? These are examples of *working memory*, or, more specifically, lapses of working memory. This type of memory relates to information we hold on to or process for about 10 to 20 seconds (that is, unless we take further steps to remember or record it). Note that working memory does double duty as both a form of memory and one of the brain's executive functions, which we'll discuss in more detail soon.

Remember our discussion in Chapter 2 related to patient H.M.? His semantic memory for information learned prior to his brain surgery was in good shape, and he could remember new names or other material for a few seconds at a time. But because his hippocampus—a structure critical for forming new episodic memories—had been removed, he was forever trapped in the brief period of working memory, being unable to lock in almost any new information for more than a few moments.

As you might imagine, working memory is strongly linked to attention, particularly sustained attention, and is also important in helping us regulate our behavior. For example, making a quick decision to avoid or opt for a slice of devil's food cake in the buffet can make a big difference in how successful a diet is. Similar to some other forms of memory, working memory can be enhanced with practice, even at the level where we see brain activity changes that correlate with improvement.

Also of note, one study found that working memory gains can occur when we affirm our core values: beliefs or principles that are particularly important to us and define who we are. While this may not immediately seem intuitive, the idea is that by explicitly clarifying our values, we can free up our ability to focus on tasks outside of ourselves more effectively and reduce the likelihood of acting outside our best interests. Affirming our values can also help with the process of adopting new habits, like exercising more often. At the end of this chapter, we'll try a related exercise with the goal of potentially improving your brain health and general wellness in this way.

COGNITIVE TRIO PART 3:
THE EXECUTIVE FUNCTIONS

Think of a company led by a visionary CEO. As an executive in charge of dozens of employees, she needs to know how to get started on important new tasks, stay goal-oriented and organized, and manage her time effectively to finish what she starts. She must regulate her own behavior well, lest she appear hotheaded, aloof, or indecisive. Problem-solving skills are critical too; any CEO worth her salt needs to create good strategies while also changing course when those strategies don't work out.

Our hypothetical CEO is tapping into her *executive functions*: a multifaceted set of cognitive skills, largely governed by the frontal lobes of the brain, that help us engage in goal-directed behavior in daily life. There are a variety of different executive functions (we'll call them EFs), some of which we'll highlight next. Importantly, research shows consistently, and convincingly, that the EFs are enhanced by lifestyle choices we make. If we improve our physical fitness, engage more with others socially, or take on mentally stimulating tasks, our EFs tend to improve. We'll get into the related details later in the book, but let's start by defining what the EFs are.

The terms *executive functions* or *executive functioning* refer to a number of different brain skills (Figure 3.2).

Like attention and memory, one can describe executive functioning in many ways. In some settings, people refer

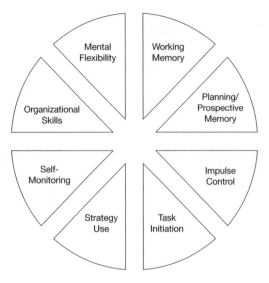

FIGURE 3.2 Types of Executive Functions

to EFs in terms of organization and time management. For example, in schools, teachers might say that a student has problems with his EF skills because he often loses his homework or procrastinates when completing assignments. In the workplace, someone with EF challenges might take a long time replying to e-mails, getting started on new tasks, or completing projects. EF difficulties in older adults could relate to problems paying bills on time or remembering to take medications. A related executive skill is called *prospective memory*: how well we remember to do something at a future time.

One EF that is particularly critical in helping us function in daily life is what neuropsychologists call *mental flexibility.*

This refers to how well we can change course with tasks, our daily schedule, and interactions when the need arises. Some students I work with struggle with mental flexibility when things don't go as planned on school-related assignments or projects. For example, they have a plan for how to finish a math assignment and get thrown for a loop when unexpected challenges arise, leading to long delays and turning homework in late. Or, consider driving to a new location. In the pre-GPS days (remember those?), we'd need to pull out a map, consider where we needed to go, and problem solve our route. Often this meant going a little out of the way to avoid traffic or other obstacles—being flexible to come up with the best solution. In general, most of us find that we need to readjust our daily plans at times, keeping our brain flexing and adjusting to unanticipated changes.

Coming back to our hypothetical CEO, what often needs to be avoided in a leadership role is appearing to fly off the handle. Managing ourselves as we respond to others—through good self-monitoring and impulse control—is critical for healthy work and personal relationships. Some are very effective at absorbing suggestions, criticism, even insults, without getting their feathers ruffled. This ability to regulate our own behavior is another important aspect of executive functioning and becomes increasingly challenging when we are, well, challenged. In a related vein, we know that stress tends to lower our tipping point, as it becomes harder to manage difficult interactions when we're generally feeling keyed up.

This brings us to a related concept discussed by psychologist Daniel Goleman: the *amygdala hijack*. When we have a stressful interaction or experience, the emerging negative feelings—generated by the brain's fire alarm, the amygdala—can overwhelm the brain, particularly the frontal lobes. Given the frontal lobes' critical role in our decision making, reasoning, planning, and concentration abilities, when they get short-circuited, we're in trouble. As emotion ramps up, blood flow to the frontal cortex diminishes, potentially resulting in impairment in EFs and other cognitive skills. While these changes are temporary, they can wreak havoc in our daily activities—it's harder to finish tasks, interact with others, and manage stress with a hijacked brain. Part of promoting brain health relates to containing and managing negative emotion, much as a skilled martial artist deflects a blow from an opponent. Otherwise, we can become distracted, forgetful, and have problems with our executive skills.

SELF-AFFIRMATION EXERCISE

We know that what's called *self-affirmation* of our personal values can be a powerful ally in the behavior-change process. There seems to be something about clarifying where we stand and what's important to us that improves our openness to learning new things. Before we move on to other topics, I'd like to introduce a related exercise that I mentioned earlier. This will also help you complete worksheets throughout the book, where you will reflect on your current values and how they are consistent with changes you'd like to make to improve your brain health. So, what I'd like you to do is take a look at the following list of concepts, attributes, and life values:

Independence   Spirituality   Tolerance   Spontaneity
Financial security   Service to others   Productivity
Community   Harmony   Accomplishment   Honesty
Optimism   Health   Kindness   Creativity   Authenticity
Sense of humor   Adaptability   Clear moral compass

Which of these are most meaningful to you? Choose six to eight of the terms above (or feel free to come up with your own) that you feel reflect your current values. Then rank-order them from most to least important in the space below.

Top Six to Eight Values
(Rank Ordered by Level of Importance to You)

1. _____

2. _____

3. _____

4. _____

5. _____

6. _____

7. _____

8. _____

Now, briefly describe why your top-ranked value is particularly meaningful to you:

_____

_____

_____

_____

_____

The exercise you just did has been associated with a number of positive outcomes, including increased ease of adopting new positive habits, better working memory, more physical activity in daily life, and improved frontal lobe functioning. I'll ask you to reflect on your values throughout the book to help clarify their personal importance and bridge the topics here to your daily activities. I hope that you'll notice various benefits to this exercise, and I suspect you will.

PART II

Cognitive Strategies and Lifestyle Activities That Boost Brain Function

4

What Strategies
Make the Most Difference?

IN THE CATEGORY OF SOMEONE MAKING LEMONADE
from lemons, Bridget had been diagnosed with multiple sclerosis (MS) a few years before I met with her for a neuropsychological evaluation. As with many people managing MS
symptoms, she had noticed some cognitive lapses in daily
life. Bridget had more problems with memory retrieval than
she used to, and she took longer to process new information
in conversation and more generally.

While the evaluation findings revealed some problems
with memory and cognitive efficiency, I also learned that she
had been ramping up her strategies to compensate for cognitive changes. She fastidiously recorded new appointments
and grocery lists in her smartphone to avoid forgetting
them. She used alarms from her phone and in her kitchen to
remind her of upcoming events or to notify her when something had cooked long enough. She also tried to remember

new names by associating them with images of people she knew with the same name. Bridget readily acknowledged her challenges, but also felt an empowering sense of control over her MS by using good strategies.

This is the first chapter in Part II of the book, which is devoted to compensatory strategies, activities, and lifestyle changes known to improve brain health and overall quality of life. This chapter will also be the first to be divided into three primary sections: "The Background Science," "The Bottom Line," and "The Brass Tacks." For "The Background Science" section, I will discuss what we know about evidence-based cognitive strategies (the "C" of the C.A.P.E. model). We'll also consider how someone like Bridget, or just about anyone for that matter, can learn to make the most of their brain health by using effective techniques for improving attention, memory, and executive functioning skills.

THE BACKGROUND SCIENCE
Real-World Strategy Use

We all probably know someone who has good memory skills: the person who remembers other people's names well, never forgets a birthday, and recalls details from parties and social events like they happened yesterday. Truth be told, there aren't many people like this. But there are some intriguing examples of people we can learn from who use powerful cognitive strategies in daily life. One is a guy named Chao Lu. Mr. Lu is a world record holder, but in a different category than most people: he holds the record for memorizing the most digits of "pi," or 3.14. (As you may know, every number after the ".14" in pi is random, and pi runs to infinity, so it's a good way to test the upper limits of memory.) In terms of his accomplishment, we're not talking about a few dozen or even a few hundred numbers (which would itself be impressive). His feat was to memorize *over 67,000 digits of pi*. Think about that for a minute. Over 67,000 digits.

It would be easy to conclude that Mr. Lu simply has a remarkable memory, better than that of just about anyone else, and call it a day. But here's what's particularly interesting: years later, when he was asked to recall as many pi digits as he could, his once impressive accomplishment was no more—he could only recall 39 digits. While nothing to scoff at, this paled in comparison to what he had once done. Upon further analysis, he was previously so good at memorizing digits because of various organizational techniques he used, and used well. These included learning two-digit groups of numbers, remembering these as words, and then creating stories and sub-stories with these words . . . hundreds and hundreds of times. Ultimately, it was his use of effective strategies that mattered more than simply having a great memory.

Another fascinating example of strategy use in the real world comes by way of South America. Experienced waiters in Buenos Aires, Argentina, are renowned for their remarkable abilities to remember complex drink and dinner orders. Some researchers found out about this and decided to pay

Buenos Aires a visit to learn more. Here's what they did: eight of them sat down at a table in some of the local hot spots and ordered a round of drinks. Waiters would then return with the scientists' order and deliver the drinks without error, as expected. After finishing their drinks (and realizing their good fortune to be getting paid to do this sort of research), the researchers ordered another round. But this time, after the waiter left the table, *they all changed seats.* Beyond a juvenile attempt to taunt the waiter, they wanted to understand whether the ability to remember a complicated drink order was tied to location. In other words, was it possible that the waiter was using visual cues or reminders to recall where the drinks should be delivered?

The scientists soon discovered that the memory capacity of the waiters wasn't so hot after all. Upon delivering the second round of drinks, the waiters made a number of errors, and were probably pretty embarrassed to have their reputations as local memory superstars tarnished. The researchers repeated the experiment with untrained waiters—those who had never waited tables before—and found that they were generally terrible at taking and correctly delivering orders. However, in the changed seat "condition" of the experiment, the novices did just as well as the trained waiters. The experienced waiters had a great strategy (tying a drink order to spatial location of the customer) that broke down when something changed. While their jig was up as a result of the scientists' ingenuity, the waiters' real-world performance—and crafty strategy use—was nevertheless impressive.

External and Internal Strategies

When we consider what cognitive strategies we can use in daily life, there are two broad categories: external and internal. An *external strategy* is one that is "external" to us that helps us manage our tasks and the settings we work and live in. In other words, these are strategies that relate to something that we can physically manipulate. Examples of external strategies abound: a smartphone (including the calendar function with alarms and vibrations as reminders), wall calendars, lists, dry-erase boards, auto-payment systems for bills, day planners, online calendars, alarm clocks, and kitchen timers. Using a pillbox to help us remember medications counts too. We can also place commonly used items—a purse, wallet, or keys—in a consistent location (like a basket by the front door) to help avoid misplacing them. Using one or more of these external strategies brings order to our environment and helps us keep track of things in daily life.

Internal strategies are mental techniques that we use in the moment to help us remember or organize new information. Rather than actually writing something down or entering it into a smartphone, internal strategies are helpful in the initial phase of learning something new. For example, mentally repeating a new friend's name a few times can help us remember it when it would be difficult to physically record it somehow. Holding a few ideas in mind using an acronym is another way that we can remember something for a brief period of time, and maybe longer. Our use of the C.A.P.E acronym certainly counts in this regard. I'll discuss a few other examples below.

As psychologist Daniel Kahneman has demonstrated in his research, too many choices are a bad thing. **So, in the subsections that follow, I've detailed a few helpful, evidence-based strategies for each part of the cognitive trio we discussed in Chapter 3: attention, memory, and executive functions.** Figure 4.1 contains examples of some of these strategies. Also, as we know from positive psychology research, it's much easier to create a positive lifestyle habit—such as using a new cognitive strategy—if we experience positive emotion while using it. So, if you try a strategy below and it results in even a brief positive emotion, a small

External strategy	Internal strategy
A paper or e-calendar/ appointment book	Verbalizing or "talking yourself through" a task
Lists with a maximum of four to five items, each of which includes task time estimates	Putting information into an acronym to help remember it later
Alarm from cell phone or kitchen timer	Attaching personal associations to new material
Having a consistent location for important items like a cell phone, wallet, or purse	Taking a mental step back when you're stuck solving a problem
Drawing something you're trying to remember	"Unitasking" instead of multitasking

FIGURE 4.1 Examples of External and Internal Strategies

success, or a mild sense of mastery over something in your day, be sure to notice this! The more you can reflect on a small improvement and feel good about it, the more you'll continue to use and benefit from the strategy.

Attention Strategies

When considering strategies we can use to enhance attention, it is important to understand that in order to remember something well, we need to focus on it first. Something I observe in many patients with cognitive complaints is that what they consider to be memory problems are actually attention lapses. Some of these lapses relate to stress and mood decline; once their stressful circumstance passes or their mood improves, they report fewer problems with memory. This change is actually seen in the science as well. Simply put, people typically report fewer memory or other cognitive problems when they feel like themselves again.

One particularly handy and evidence-based internal strategy to improve attention is verbalizing a task, or literally saying out loud what you are doing, step by step. Another way to think about this is as if you were a "play-by-play announcer" at a sports game. There seems to be something about describing our process aloud that allows the brain to focus better on the task at hand and reduce the effects of background distractions.

It takes some practice to get the hang of self-talk while completing a chore, work task, or something you're doing in school. Initially, the idea is to clarify the overall plan for completing the task. Then, while proceeding through the task, say out loud what you're doing each step of the way. As you practice, you can subvocalize each step—saying each one under your breath—and then eventually fade your speech to silence while mentally continuing the process. There are simple ways to practice; for example, while cleaning the dishes, talk your way through each glass, dish, and piece of silverware you're cleaning. While doing the laundry, describe—out loud, but under your breath—each item you're removing from the dryer and folding. Over time, the process of verbalizing a task can become second nature, and you'll likely find that you're able to concentrate better on a wide variety of tasks.

A great external strategy to sharpen our attention on tasks is a simple one: a distraction notepad. This comes from the research on ADHD, where managing distractions is of paramount importance. Here's the idea: when working on a task at school, at work, or at home, we often have distracting thoughts (How did my sports team do last night? What time do I need to pick my daughter up after soccer practice? Is my dry cleaning done today?). Rather than respond to the thought (for example, checking a sports website for the team's score), write the thought down on a sticky note or in a specific notepad for this purpose. By doing this, the thought is effectively neutralized—it's been recorded for later action—and you can stay focused on the current task.

In our increasingly high-tech world, distractions are everywhere. Cell phones, tablets, social media, the Internet always at our beck and call . . . it's certainly hard to focus effectively when our environments are so saturated with options to throw us off task. As a related external attention-enhancing strategy, try to be deliberate with your media use. Are there times when you don't need to get breaking news alerts on your phone or computer? Do you get a ping every time an e-mail or text message comes through? Take control by turning off these notifications or, better yet, turn off your phone and close your e-mail program when you need to focus intently on the task at hand. Use social media mindfully as a reward for completing a daily task rather than letting it intrude upon your process.

Attention and Flow A well-researched and powerful state of mind relates to our discussion of attention-boosting strategies in daily life: *flow*. In particular, the *flow state*, as discussed by psychologist Mihaly Csikszentmihalyi, involves deep and sustained focus on an activity or task. It's when we feel totally absorbed in what we're doing, so much so that we lose track of time. Flow is a very desirable state to be in: productivity and enjoyment go hand in hand, and the workday flies by without thinking about it. Being engrossed in non-work pursuits, such as playing music, creating visual or other art, or involvement in athletics, are other examples of flow.

Consider the actress who is completely committed to her role, thoroughly convincing the audience that she *is* the character being played, resulting in a high-caliber performance. Or the computer programmer who is able to focus intently for hours at a time creating new software. Perhaps it's the downhill skier who is performing at the top of her game, winning a race by a few hundredths of a second because she was so focused on her line and the nuances of the course. We can also think of the weekend hobbyist, crafting a perfect birdhouse over many hours to the eventual delight of grateful blue jays.

The flow state occurs under several conditions and using certain strategies. These include having a specific goal, being motivated to take on a task, and having previous experience with the task. It's also important that we have the resources we need. These might include a quiet room, necessary materials like a well-operating computer, and perhaps a style of music that you just listen to while completing similar tasks. As you might imagine, some things can prevent us from getting into a flow state, including a less-than-ideal environment, excess stress, and interpersonal conflicts.

The flow state occurs when we've got a good balance between what the task demands are and the skills we bring to bear to complete it. Feeling unchallenged by something that's easy for us results in boredom. Feeling too challenged without the right skill set leads to anxiety. Can you think of a time when you were functioning at a peak performance level? Consider what was going on right before you started the task, what it felt like to be using your skills well despite being challenged, and what the end result or outcome was. Finding that state whenever possible is desirable for any activity, and is another great way to promote brain health.

Memory Strategies

As we get into middle age and beyond, we're less effective at committing new information to memory, so we need to be more active in the learning process. As one example, how many times have you forgotten someone's name after being introduced? (Me too.) Your focus is on the person for a brief moment, and then a conversational thread takes you elsewhere. All of a sudden, you have no idea what his or her name is! Here's something you can try the next time you meet someone. A good first step is to introduce yourself after saying that person's name first. For example: "Hi, Mike, I'm John." As you repeat their name, your brain responds by building neural connections linking their name and face. This increases the chances of remembering their name later in the interaction, the next day, and beyond.

A powerful next step is to attach some sort of a personal association to their name and relate this information to something you already know. One way to do this is to come up with a mental image of the new person standing next to someone you already know with the same name. Coming back to "Mike," let's say you used to work with or went to school with someone named Mike—someone you've known for years. Now create an image in your mind of the "new" Mike standing next to the "old" Mike, perhaps shaking hands, talking to each other, tossing a hot coal back and forth . . . you get the idea. At some level, the goofier the mental image, the better. In turn, you have helped your brain make an even deeper connection to the new name you just learned, boosting the chances of remembering Mike's name the next time you see him. You can also practice this strategy at home—perhaps by trying to learn the name of someone in the news, a sportscaster, or a cooking show host—to get yourself in the habit. In a way, you have a private "laboratory" to work on improving your memory strategies any time you'd like.

This process is also called *elaboration*—creating a broader context for new things you're learning—and is particularly effective if you want to learn and retain information better. A related strategy is what's called *spaced practice*. This is an internal strategy where you initially learn some new material (perhaps content from a class you've taken or something you've recently read) and then let some time elapse before coming back to the material and reviewing it. The idea is to take a break, engage in another activity, take a nap, or even turn in for the night. Then afterward, come back to the content you've learned and retest yourself.

As Peter Brown and his colleagues write in their helpful book, *Make It Stick*, this strategy is much more effective than the traditional "cramming" strategy that many students use. The latter might help you do better on a test the next day, but the inevitable mental toilet flush will likely follow soon thereafter, taking you back to square one with little if any longer-term retention.

Another internal strategy you can use is one that should already be familiar: putting information into some sort of meaningful structure or "package" that can be easily retrieved later. Much of this book relates to the C.A.P.E.

model, which refers to key ways to promote brain health. You're probably able to define the four parts of this acronym at this point (cognitive strategies, activity engagement, prevention of cognitive problems, and education about the brain), suggesting that you've already been using this strategy. Maybe there are other common ideas, tasks, or bits of information in your own life that you can create an easily remembered acronym for too.

A simple but very effective external memory strategy is *drawing* what you're trying to remember. Some innovative studies have looked at how drawing something compares to other memory techniques, and it turns out that at least for some types of information, this is a great way to go. One study compared different strategies that might help people remember a list of words—things like writing the words down or creating mental images of words—and found that drawing words was the winner. Even if the researchers made the list longer or gave people less time to remember words, it didn't matter; drawing still helped people remember better. One application in daily life might be to make a quick sketch of items to be picked up at the grocery store, or to draw a scene related to a period of U.S. history when studying for a test. You don't have to be a great artist! The process of merely drawing what you're trying to remember is what counts.

Executive Functioning Strategies

Many of my patients with cognitive concerns report problems remembering mundane but important tasks in daily life: appointments at work, school, or with doctors; paying bills on time; where they parked their car at a shopping mall or at the supermarket; where they placed items like keys or a smartphone. Folks also frequently report having word-finding difficulties in conversation. These, in fact, are common complaints in the general population. The science indicates that these are the types of problems people report at high levels: one large study found that over half of middle-aged men and about two-thirds of women describe having memory difficulties.

Fortunately, these are the types of concerns that can be managed using straightforward external strategies that I would put in the *executive functioning* category. This is because they involve ways to plan, organize information, and manage time, ultimately resulting in better ability to remember things.

For those interested in "old school" techniques, consistently using an appointment book or wall calendar is a great way to go, particularly for remembering future meetings. We all live busy lives, and remembering an appointment weeks or months away is difficult to do spontaneously for most people (probably even for our memory champion, Chao Lu). Using organizational habits and strategies to help with planning for future events can make a huge difference.

Having an appointment book that is compact, easy to use (with days and weeks laid out in a way that works well for you), stylish (however you define that), and always nearby can help prevent a missed meeting with a friend or colleague. Some people prefer using a smartphone or online calendar to do the same thing. These strategies are helpful because they provide reminders through multiple sensory channels: a visual reminder by seeing the event listed, an auditory reminder with an alarm chime, and even a tactile reminder with a vibration. They also reduce stress by getting pressing details out of our minds and onto a page (paper or electronic), where they can be considered and acted upon when the time is right.

How about misplacing items in daily life? Do you tend to misplace your keys, purse, or wallet? Placing objects in a consistent location at home or at work is the best way to manage these lapses. For example, using a basket by the front door for this purpose can be helpful. While this can take some time to become habitual, eventually you'll find that misplacing daily items will happen considerably less often. High-tech strategies can help here too. There are small devices you can buy that go on your keychain ring and can be linked to a phone app, allowing you to ping the location of your keys using GPS. Pretty cool for those interested in stepping up their game a little using technology.

Another external executive function strategy is recording information effectively for "acute" tasks. These are tasks you need to complete on any given day and require short-term planning to manage effectively. It goes without saying that making a list is the way to go here; however, not all lists are created equal. A list of many items—while helpful as a separate master task list—can be overwhelming and counterproductive.

Ideally, task lists that are being used in any given part of a day have no more than four to five items. By using lists that are brief like this, you increase the chances of completing the list (and crossing off each task feels pretty good), leading to a sense of accomplishment and mastery. An important add-on for lists is to estimate how long you think each task will take. While your estimate may be off a bit, this process nevertheless helps mentally frame your efforts, time-wise, and provides a more realistic sense of your ability to complete tasks in the time you have. For example, a list of five items to work on in the first half of the day might look like this:

- Complete expense report (60 minutes)
- Call colleague to discuss collaboration next month (15 minutes)
- Call son's teacher to schedule parent–teacher conference (10 minutes)
- Pay electric and phone bills (10 minutes)

It's clear that the expense report is the most time-consuming item on the list. This should probably be tackled first given that it will take the longest (and maybe longer than we estimate). The other tasks are quicker and can probably be fit in later in the morning. There's always some wiggle room with time estimates, and it's important to leave some buffer for unexpected interruptions (a colleague stops by your office to chat; you get a call at home from a relative you haven't heard from in a long time; you decide to get up and walk around to avoid being sedentary for too long). This process can ultimately lead you to gain more control over your schedule and, in turn, use your executive functions advantageously to improve your productivity.

One important aspect of executive functioning we discussed in Chapter 3 is what neuropsychologists call *mental flexibility*. This essentially refers to how well we can change course when needed in daily life. When was the last time that you had something in your schedule you needed to change? Or worked on a project at home, where your original plan unexpectedly needed to be revised? Or were in a conversation that morphed into a new and unfamiliar topic, and you needed to regroup and follow along? We all need to be flexible with our activities and plans; this is simply part of being human. Striving to be flexible is also an important aspect of brain fitness.

One key way to promote mental flexibility: do a quick self-monitoring exercise in moments when you feel you're not progressing on a task the way you'd like. Take a mental step back (what I like to call the "40,000 foot" perspective, as if looking at your situation from a distance), take a few deep breaths (to help your brain avoid an amygdala hijack due to frustration and anxiety), and ask yourself whether there is something you could do differently in this situation. And, do a self-check to see if you've decided on a plan of attack too quickly. While it can be helpful to think on our feet and make a quick decision, it can be just as important to take our time and consider various options before committing to a strategy.

Chris was a middle-aged patient I worked with who mentioned that he had struggled to find the right health insurance plan. One plan offered some benefits that were appealing, and it was fairly inexpensive, but he hadn't appreciated the high deductible he'd have to pay before benefits kicked in. Just before committing to the plan, his wife realized the considerable risk of paying far more for the deductible than was necessary given their health issues. They ended up going with a plan that cost a little more on a monthly basis—but had a much lower deductible—that was more in line with their needs. Taking a step back to see the broader financial implications made the difference between a well-reasoned decision and one that could have broken the bank. Being flexible paid off, literally and figuratively.

One other executive function strategy to mention relates to how we proceed through a task. As we discussed earlier, research shows that multitasking—working on a few things simultaneously—causes us to make more mistakes, slow down, and be less productive. A more effective way to go is what's called *unitasking*—taking on one task, completing it, and then moving to the next one. This way, you're working with your brain rather than against it.

An add-on to this process is to unitask by starting with the most important task and then moving to the next most important one. While it might seem easier and more appealing to work on something that will only take a few minutes, this can take us off course and ultimately interfere with more critical tasks. Distractions during the day are part and parcel of all of our lives. This is why working on the most important task first will improve your overall workflow and lead to more time later in the day to manage smaller things.

And just to reinforce an earlier point: it's important to reflect on your emotion during and after using cognitive strategies discussed here and more generally. Do you feel an uptick in your feelings when you've successfully recorded a future event, planned for it, and arrived on time? Are your efforts to unitask leading to less stress and tension in the moment and day to day? The more positive the experience, the more likely you'll build the strategy into your routine and feel satisfied with how you're taking care of your responsibilities.

THE BOTTOM LINE

So, summarizing a few key points from this chapter:

- As you consider strategies that can help you focus, remember, and stay organized in daily life, use a balance of strategies that are *internal* (self-generated) and *external* (something tangible or in your environment, like a calendar or sticky notes).
- For promoting attention, try to verbalize or "talk yourself through" tasks.

- To improve memory, attach personal associations to new information you're trying to learn.

- Add structure to new information, such as placing material into an easily remembered acronym (like C.A.P.E. for cognitive strategies, activity engagement, prevention of cognitive problems, and education about the brain).

- Keep important items (like keys or your smartphone) in a consistent place at home and at work.

- Keep lists to four or five total items, and include time estimates for how long each item will take to complete.

- Avoid multitasking and instead try to unitask.

- When you get stuck trying to figure something out, take a mental step back to view the problem from a distance, take a few deep breaths, and ask yourself if there are any other options at hand that might be better than the one you're using.

- Reflect on positive emotions (even brief ones) you've felt while using a cognitive strategy in daily life. This increases the chances of the strategy becoming part of your routine.

- Getting into a flow state is an ideal way to channel cognitive skills positively and increase productivity. Strategies to do this include preparing well before you start a task at work or at home, being in an environment with all the resources you need, and having a positive and engaged attitude.

THE BRASS TACKS:
PERSONAL STRATEGIC PLANNING TO
IMPROVE MY COGNITIVE STRATEGY USE

Current strategies I typically use each day (or at least a few times per week): _____

_____

_____

When I use these strategies: _____

_____

_____

Factors that get in the way of me using these strategies more:

_____

_____

_____

Top two barriers that make it hard for me to use effective cognitive strategies: _____

_____

_____

What I can do to overcome barrier #1:

_____

_____

_____

What I can do to overcome barrier #2:

_____

_____

_____

Small steps I can take to use strategies (even a little bit more) this week: _____

_____

_____

Small steps I can take to use strategies (even a little bit more) this month: _____

_____

_____

Strategy-use goals I have for myself over the next 3 months:

_____

_____

_____

Strategy-use goals I have for myself over the next 6 months:

_____

_____

_____

Things I've learned from this chapter that could help me use strategies more often: _____

_____

_____

How using additional strategies is consistent with my current values (the ones I indicated at the end of Chapter 3):

_____

_____

_____

5

What Does Exercise
Do for the Brain?

STEVE TENDED TO DO THE RIGHT THINGS FOR HIS body and brain. He exercised regularly, ate well (with the help of his wife, an excellent cook), and tried to stay mentally stimulated through reading and perfecting his guitar skills. I saw him when he was in his late fifties after he and his wife noticed that his memory was starting to slip. He was still functioning well in daily life, but the memory lapses were becoming more inconvenient and embarrassing. His neuropsychological testing scores revealed some problems learning new verbal information, such as new stories or a word list, but he otherwise looked just fine. In fact, he was fairly strong in some areas. His overall pattern indicated that he had mild cognitive impairment (MCI), and I recommended that he return every 1 to 2 years for reevaluations to keep an eye on his cognitive status.

There was continued evidence of memory problems

each time I saw him, but he did not develop more troubling signs of dementia. Despite the fact that roughly 10% of individuals with MCI progress to dementia every year, Steve was beating the odds. When I asked him about exercise, he would consistently tell me: "After what you told me about exercise and the brain, I wasn't going to let that slide." He continued his routine of 30 to 45 minutes on the treadmill almost every day, and I told him that his level of activity was likely playing a positive role in promoting his brain functioning and cognitive skills.

THE BACKGROUND SCIENCE

In our C.A.P.E. model of brain health, the "A" stands for *activity engagement*, and three types of activity are referenced by the model. Over the next few chapters, we'll consider these three types of activity: physical activity and exercise; social activity and engagement; and mental or intellectual activity. **This chapter focuses on the importance of physical activity for the brain and cognition.**

First off, if you don't exercise that much, you're not alone. Surveys on levels of physical activity in the general population are sobering. Only about 20% of adults and elders exercise at levels recommended by the U.S. Department of Health and Human Services and the American Heart Association (at least 30 minutes of aerobic activity 5 days per week, and muscle strengthening 2+ days per week). Some of us might find that level of exercise a bit unrealistic, especially if we're not currently very active. Fortunately, we know that exercising 20 to 30 minutes per day—even if we just take brisk walks—has a powerful impact on the brain. We'll discuss this more later.

We also find that beyond being physically active in a traditional sense, many people sit far too much and stand far too little. Recent research has clarified that around the world—in 54 separate countries—excessive sitting during the day is linked to an increased likelihood of death after accounting for other causes. Who thought something so seemingly benign could be so dangerous? Another study found that the more hours per day you spend sitting, the smaller your medial temporal lobe tends to be. This part of the brain is particularly important for learning and memory, so research findings like this are concerning if you tend to be sedentary most of the time (especially at work). It seems that getting up and moving around, even for brief periods of time, really makes a difference for overall health *and* for brain health.

What do we mean when we refer to "exercise"? While we intuitively understand this term, there are many activities that fall under the broad category of exercise. Walking, jogging, dancing, cycling, swimming, skiing, snowboarding, mountain biking, and hiking are only a few. As long as we're sweating and our heart is beating harder than usual, it counts. The other thing to keep in mind is that combining physical activity with something mentally or socially engaging is particularly powerful for the brain: think tennis, racquetball, or going on a brisk walk with a friend or coworker.

Why is it that people don't seem to exercise much? We can think of a few common barriers that interfere with getting more exercise:

- *Environmental barriers.* Some people live in climates that aren't very conducive to getting out and regularly engaging in outdoor activities like hiking, walking, cycling, or playing tennis or other sports. Late fall through spring tends to be a time to stay hunkered down to avoid the cold, resulting in setbacks to our efforts to exercise more in warmer months. The opposite also applies: when it's too hot or humid, it becomes easy to justify staying inside and waiting for a cooler day to get out and move.
- *Time barriers.* This is one we can all relate to: the sense that there just isn't enough time in the day to exercise. Most people feel chronically busy, if not consistently behind in their work and home lives. Adding in another activity such as exercise just seems unrealistic.
- *Misconceptions about exercise.* It can be difficult to exercise consistently when we worry that brief periods of activity will make us sore later or believe that exercise will only benefit us if it's intense and lengthy.
- *Health concerns.* Some are concerned that due to medical conditions such as heart disease, obesity, or chronic pain, exercise might have a negative impact and should be avoided.
- *Minimal or inconsistent support from others related to exer-*

cise. Starting an exercise program of any sort on your own can be very difficult, particularly if you receive mixed or even negative messages. Hearing from a friend or healthcare professional that you "should exercise more"—especially without any meaningful suggestions on how to actually do this—can be frustrating, embarrassing, even demoralizing.

While these barriers to activity can all be justified at some level, they can also impede even subtle shifts in ramping up exercise that can be healthy for your body *and* your mind. By exploring and challenging our own beliefs that get in the way of physical activity, we can often find excuses *to* exercise. Environmental barriers can be managed for many people by joining an inexpensive gym or recreation center, going on walks in a shopping mall during particularly cold or warm days, using a stationary bike, or walking or jogging on a treadmill.

Time barriers can also be seen as opportunities; for example, instead of parking close to the building where you work or do errands, park on the other side of the parking lot. Try the stairs instead of taking the elevator. The extra few minutes of walking time from these small shifts can gradually add up, especially if done multiple times per day. Importantly, exercise can be just as good for the brain and body if it's broken up into small chunks (say, 5 to 10 minutes at a time).

Misconceptions about exercise may be believable enough

that they interfere with getting active, but it's important to challenge them too; for example, you don't have to force the "no pain, no gain" workouts to experience brain-related benefits, and exercise is important for everyone, including those with chronic health problems. While it's always good to check with your healthcare provider about a new exercise routine, most medical problems do not preclude exercise. If anything, exercise tends to reduce medical symptoms and improve quality of life regardless of where you may fall on the health–illness spectrum.

General Benefits of Exercise

To play the devil's advocate, what's all the hype about exercise? We all know at some level that being active and getting our heart rate up is a good idea. But what is actually happening in our body, particularly in our brain, to suggest that we should prioritize exercise on a regular basis?

First, the science indicates that exercise has a number of direct and indirect effects on the body's cardiovascular system. We know that exercise reduces high blood pressure, which in turn lessens the chances of sustaining small lesions in the brain. These lesions occur with some frequency in those with poorly managed hypertension and can lead to cognitive problems, as we'll discuss in Chapter 11. More generally, about 30 minutes per day is ideal to maintain good cardiovascular health, but even small amounts of exercise are helpful. So, if you're not a marathon runner, long-distance cyclist, or competitive swimmer, have no fear: any exercise is good for you.

We also see a significant reduction in two major causes of medical complications and death—heart disease and diabetes—in those who exercise. Working out reduces our chance of minor or catastrophic strokes, either of which can lead to a variety of changes in our memory, other thinking skills, mobility, and overall quality of life. Exercise also helps us sleep better and keep our weight down. We all experience varying levels of stress, and physical activity allows us to manage stress better and helps our mood stay more positive and less grouchy.

When we think specifically about positive effects of exercise on the brain, there are a number of additional benefits. Many of these benefits are summed up by a related adage: *What's good for your heart is good for your brain.* So, activity or dietary changes that are known to improve heart health work for the brain too. We also know that there is simply no better intervention to date that impacts the brain so profoundly and completely as exercise. We'll discuss some related details next.

How Exercise Boosts Brain Structure and Function

Perhaps the most exciting development in the science of exercise and the brain—and one that both surprised scientists and upended decades of knowledge about how the brain operates—is the finding that *exercise grows new neurons*. This brain benefit is a fairly recent discovery, and flies in the face of the long-held axiom that the brain is set in stone after early development. Indeed, in the not-too-distant past, it was believed that we were born with a finite amount of neurons that were preordained in terms of overall quantity and features. Neurons didn't grow or change throughout life—certainly not in a positive direction—and merely faded away as we aged. A fairly bleak portrait of the brain, to be sure. We now know that neurons grow in response to exercise in two critically important brain regions—the hippocampus and the frontal cortex—that are associated with learning new material, solving problems, processing information, and some types of attention. Simply put, having more neurons improves our cognitive power and efficiency; the more we have, the stronger our memory, executive functioning, and processing skills are. **Let's dive into some of the revolutionary science that clarifies how we can ramp up our own *neurogenesis,* or neuron growth.**

In one of the early studies to demonstrate how the brain responds to exercise, people were asked to exercise for a year, 3 days per week, for 40 minutes per workout. After a few weeks getting up to speed, they were asked to walk at a moderate rate—at 60% to 75% of their maximum heart rate—for the rest of the study. Note that this was an inactive group before the study began: they hadn't exercised for more than 30 minutes in the previous 6 months. That's pretty sedentary.

About halfway through the study, and then after a year, the researchers used neuroimaging to determine brain-related changes. What they found was remarkable: compared to a control group that was only stretching, the brisk walkers had literally grown their brains by exercising. In particular, the participants' hippocampus had grown at a level that essentially erased the expected 1% to 2% decline in volume during that time. Importantly, the control group showed this typical annual reduction in hippocampal volume, indicating that exercise had done something powerful for the "treatment" group.

More recent research has supported this earlier work. For example, one study asked a group of previously sedentary people to walk, jog, or ride a stationary bike 30 to 60 minutes at a time, 3 days per week, for 6 months. The trainers working with the study participants gradually increased their heart rate to 80% of maximum rate, so they were pushing things pretty hard. At the completion of the study, compared to a control group who just did stretching and muscle toning, the exercisers showed significantly better thinking skills on a global level (including improved memory, processing speed, and executive functions). In addition, *the more their fitness improved during the study, the bigger their hippocampus got.* These findings show us that exercise is a fantastic way to ramp up one's brain plasticity; that is, the brain's tendency to change in response to stimulation or activity.

Beyond the addition of new neurons and growth of the brain, we also see powerful effects of exercise on multiple neurochemicals in the brain. One area that's received a lot of attention is how neuroprotective factors such as brain-derived neurotrophic factor (BDNF) respond to exercise. BDNF is an important compound within the brain because of its role in supporting the health of the billions of neurons we have. Indeed, BDNF helps new neurons develop, and it also helps existing neurons communicate better. Research also indicates that BDNF is strongly associated with our ability to focus, learn, and remember new things.

One of the interesting things about BDNF is that exercise promotes its availability in the brain in three ways. First, single bouts of exercise boost BDNF levels, and this increase is associated with improvement in multiple cognitive skills, including memory and executive functioning. It also seems to be the case that a single period of exercise impacts BDNF levels more positively in people who are physically fit. Further, people who exercise consistently have a higher concentration of this neurotrophin at rest. All of these observations indicate that exercise has a powerful effect on the brain at the level of brain structures all the way down to the basic chemistry of the brain.

An area within neuroscience that has been looked at recently is how markers of inflammation in the body affect brain structure and function. Inflammation occurs after acute injuries, which is a normal biological response. However, chronic inflammation in the body and brain can lead to more significant medical issues. Some research has even highlighted a connection between inflammation and Alzhei-

mer's disease. Fortunately, there's evidence that higher physical fitness and exercise levels reduce inflammation, and this
reduction is associated with better cognitive functioning.
Physical activity also helps support and grow the vasculature
of the brain—the vessels that carry life-sustaining, oxygen-
rich blood to all the brain's various nooks and crannies.

Exercise additionally decreases the chance of developing
Alzheimer's disease and other forms of dementia. In fact,
physical inactivity is a "modifiable risk factor" that is associated with more cases of Alzheimer's disease in the U.S.
than any other factor we can potentially control (such as diabetes, obesity, smoking, and high blood pressure). Beyond
reducing the risk of dementia on a general level, a key finding in the science is that the risk gets progressively lower
the more types of physical activity you engage in. In other
words, if you're into cross-training, your brain is reaping
the rewards! The research supporting the protective effects
of exercise on dementia prevention is compelling, and we'll
discuss more of the details later in the chapter.

Types and Intensity of Exercise and Brain Health

Which types of activity matter the most? **Fundamentally,
just about any form of exercise or physical activity is good for
the brain.** The most frequently studied types of exercise are
walking and jogging, probably because these activities are
easier to quantify in scientific experiments. Research looking at the effects of walking on the brain generally shows

that you don't need to jog, run, or do marathons to grow neurons in important brain regions.

A study conducted a few years ago looked at the effects of low-intensity walking—just regular, daily walking—on the size of the brain's memory-critical hippocampus. A group of older adults was asked to wear a device for about a week that counted daily steps and periods of continuous activity that lasted at least 10 minutes. The participants also underwent brain scans to see if their activity levels were related to the size of a few different brain areas.

The findings indicated that for every 1,000 steps walked per day, the participants' hippocampus tended to be a little bit bigger. The pattern was similar for every 10-minute interval of additional walking—again, more exercise equaled a larger hippocampus—though the time spent exercising was less impressive than the total steps taken. These findings held true after accounting for factors such as age, education level, and cardiovascular problems, all of which can influence results in these types of studies. Curiously, the findings applied to women but not men; some studies, like this one, have found that exercise might have stronger effects on women's brains.

Other research has found that walking 6 to 9 miles per week is linked to greater volume in multiple brain areas, especially the frontal lobes and temporal lobes. So, walking about a mile a day has measurable and significant effects on how much overall brain tissue you have at your disposal. While sustained walking or running may have the best effects on the brain, recent research has found that other types of activity help the brain too. For example, yoga can promote richer connections throughout the brain and improve memory, and tai chi can enhance attention, memory, and language skills. There's also evidence that aqua aerobics can improve working memory and some types of attention, and cycling boosts verbal and visual memory, particularly right after a cycling session.

How intense should exercise be to maximize brain-related benefits? Overall, moderately intense exercise is particularly helpful, and much of what we know about the brain-exercise connection stems from studies where this intensity level is emphasized. We also find in the science that the relationship between exercise and cardiovascular health (and likely, by extension, brain health) appears to be "curvilinear": both low and high intensity exercise are better for your heart than non-exercise, but moderately intense activity is the sweet spot for heart-related benefits. By the way, "moderate" exercise refers to about a 5 or 6 on a 0 to 10 scale of exertion, where "0" means standing still and "10" represents running full blast. A 5 to 6 activity level might include hiking, a brisk walk, biking at a moderate pace, or swimming laps more than casually but not at race speed.

We also tend to see a *dose–response relationship* between exercise and cognitive gains. In other words, the higher your exercise "dose"—one refreshing walk for 20 minutes versus two to three similar walks in a week—the more your brain reaps the rewards. For example, one study found that walking or jogging 75 minutes per week ramped up attention and visual–spatial skills, and doubling the workout time improved some abilities even more. Other research has found that from our teens to our seventies, exercising up to 2 hours per week benefits executive functioning and, to a lesser extent, memory. These benefits are even more robust when people exercise more than that.

A massive recent study—involving over 100,000 people across 20 countries—further clarified the dose–response relationship with regard to exercise. The researchers followed people over an 8-year period, and found that those who worked out fairly regularly showed better memory and language skills than those who never exercised. A particularly compelling finding from the study was that the more physically active people were, the better they performed on cognitive tests. It also seemed to be the case that people who weren't very active at the beginning of the study but got moving later showed significant improvement in their thinking skills. The take-home message from this research is that any exercise at all is good for your brain, and nudging yourself to do a little more is even better.

It's also important to point out that the amount of time you exercise doesn't have to be all at once. In other words, if you're trying to exercise for 20 minutes per day, you can break this into two 10-minute exercise sessions (a few walks, climbing stairs at the office, and so on). Even though many of our days tend to be very busy, splitting exercise into smaller chunks makes it easier to fit in a mini-workout. In a related vein, if you've only got a few minutes for exercise, you may still notice a brief boost in brainpower; individual exercise sessions have been found to temporarily improve our focus and executive functioning skills.

Another way to think about exercise time: How much exercise do I need to engage in before I notice lasting cognitive benefits? A reasonable answer comes from a study that reviewed about 100 clinical trials that were done with people aged 60 or older. Most of the science that was reviewed involved aerobic activity (usually, walking) or aerobic workouts combined with resistance training. The key finding: less than 52 hours didn't have much of an effect, but 52 hours or more did. There were particular benefits for executive functions and processing speed with this amount of exercise, and fewer gains for memory. Each exercise session across studies was usually about an hour, and studies in the review typically lasted around 6 months. But again, the total time exercised over weeks and months mattered more. Ultimately, it may take a while to experience noticeable cognitive improvement from exercise, but there's now convincing evidence indicating that it will happen with time and effort (and a little patience).

One approach to exercise that's getting more scientific and popular attention is high-intensity interval training (which I'll call HIIT). Briefly, HIIT involves brief periods of high-intensity exercise that alternate with brief periods of light exercise. Practically speaking, think running at nearly full speed for a minute or two followed by walking for another minute or two, and then repeating this cycle a few times.

Beyond improving one's fitness level, there's also some evidence that HIIT sessions have benefits for the brain. In particular, people tend to process information more efficiently and be less error-prone after a period of HIIT. HIIT may also boost executive functioning skills for a longer period than moderate exercise after single workout sessions. One study found that a session of HIIT led to better mental flexibility, and that this improvement was linked to more BDNF. As an added benefit, HIIT has also been found to enhance physical fitness better than moderate exercise.

It's important to reiterate that most of the research on exercise and the brain has involved light to moderate activity levels, both of which we know are really good for the brain. Given that HIIT is a relative newcomer to this area of research, it remains unclear whether HIIT provides more ongoing benefit for cognition than less intense exercise. Stay tuned, as the initial evidence looks promising.

Reaping the Benefits of Midlife Fitness

We know that beginning to exercise at any point in life is very much worth doing. People who have been sedentary but begin to work out in their later years (even in their eighties) experience important health benefits, including positive brain changes. Of particular importance for individuals in midlife: *our fitness levels during that life phase predict our brain health 20 to 30 years later*. Multiple studies have shown that the more fit we are in midlife, the lower our chances are of developing dementia. Fitness in middle age is more generally linked to a better working brain decades from now. In fact, any level of physical activity is associated with a lower risk of cognitive impairment down the road. Even in the near term, stronger cardiovascular fitness in middle age is associated with more brain volume and more robust connections throughout the brain 5 years later.

One of the longest studies examining exercise and the brain—a time span of up to 44 years—was recently conducted with a large sample of Swedish women. Their physical fitness was assessed in midlife, and then they were followed over the ensuing decades to determine whether and when they met clinical criteria for dementia. In another evidence-based plug for the importance of physical activity, women who were most physically fit at midlife were much less likely to develop dementia—88% *less likely*—than those who were moderately fit. For very fit women who eventually developed Alzheimer's or other forms of dementia, the dementia occurred about 10 years later than in those with lower levels of fitness. We think a lot about planning for the future in our society, particularly in terms of having enough money and resources for retirement. Another priority certainly should be investing in midlife physical fitness given the eventual payoff many years down the road.

It is also increasingly apparent that the earlier we consider how to improve brain health, the more we benefit in the long run. Along these lines, recent research followed a group of over 3,000 children and adolescents for 31 years. Individuals with early-life high blood pressure, high cholesterol, and a smoking habit showed significantly worse learning and memory skills in midlife compared to those in better health. Importantly, this was after accounting for adulthood medical issues, suggesting that poorer childhood health had lasting effects on cognition decades later.

The executive functions of the brain—skills that include planning, time management, working memory, and task shifting—also really respond to exercise throughout the life span, including in young and middle-aged adults. For example, we know that exercise increases BDNF, the important neuroprotective compound we considered earlier. Some work has shown that there is less BDNF in the brains of middle-aged adults who have excessive fatty tissue in the abdominal area. In turn, this biological profile of sorts is also associated with reduced executive functioning. By extension, more exercise can help enhance executive function skills through increasing BDNF levels in the brain. Simply put, it's never too late to start exercising more regularly to boost cardiovascular and brain health, although fitness in midlife is particularly important.

Maintaining the Exercise Habit

So how do we start exercising, and how do we keep it up? In addition to the worksheet at the end of the chapter, which will allow you to work through some factors on your end, there are a few other things we know can help. People who maintain a consistent exercise habit are often internally motivated to do so, but also tend to have a friend who is pretty active. This suggests that spending more time with friends who exercise could have what some researchers call a "contagious" effect; in other words, being around others who like to exercise may shift your perspective and motivate you to exercise more too. Even better, getting into an exercise routine with a buddy will likely keep the habit in place (and give you a chance to socialize at the same time, an added bonus that we'll discuss in Chapter 6).

The form of activity you engage in also needs to be enjoyable. Some people really try to embody the "no pain, no gain" philosophy . . . and then burn out and become sedentary again. Maybe it's committing to a 15-minute lunchtime walk a few days a week, dusting off the mountain bike and going on a weekly ride, or finding your goggles and jumping into the pool again to do some laps. At some level, you need to enjoy both the process of exercising *and* the type of exercise itself.

In addition, what you look at while exercising really seems to matter. Pleasant scenery and being outside tend to motivate people to be more active. I would also argue that while using a stationary device like a treadmill, elliptical, or stationary cycle is inherently pretty boring for most people, watching an engaging show would probably count in the pleasant scenery category. Some people reserve "guilty pleasure" shows or series for the treadmill—ones that you don't watch at other times—as an incentive to work out.

Building any sort of habit needs to become a priority. With exercise, scheduling a few blocks each week that are dedicated to working out—no exceptions—can be a great way to move forward. Think about it: If you have a meeting with your boss or an important client, do you consider this an optional activity? When physical activity is prioritized definitively in this way, the chances of building it into your life increase quite a bit.

Other factors to consider: convenience and cost. Exercise should be relatively easy to do. Getting to where you exercise shouldn't be complicated; walking around your neighborhood or outside your office at lunchtime are both simple ways to get some time in. If you need to drive a ways to get to the gym (or to a distant trail for hiking or mountain biking), this could interfere with making the activity a consistent habit. You also should avoid paying an arm and a leg for physical activity. Steep gym membership costs can be a real deterrent for many people, whereas no-cost walks, jogs, or biking sessions are a great way to go. Gyms usually offer day passes, where for a relatively low fee you can go for a swim or other workout to spice things up from time to time without committing to a monthly fee.

THE BOTTOM LINE

Here's the bottom line for exercise and its effects on the brain and our cognitive abilities:

- Exercise benefits brain structure and function in multiple ways.
- Any type of exercise is good for the heart and brain, although most of the research to date on the brain–exercise relationship has examined the effects of casual or brisk walking.
- Physical activity helps the brain work better in those with or without medical conditions and reduces the risk of developing dementia and other chronic health problems.
- Exercising 75 minutes per week (about 10 to 15 minutes per day) leads to some brain and cognitive benefits.
- Exercising 150+ minutes per week (20 to 30 minutes per day) is even better for the brain and cognition.
- Moderately paced exercise (a 5 to 6 rating on a 0 to 10 scale of minimum to maximum exertion) seems particularly good for the brain, but high-intensity exercise can also be helpful.
- Adding a social component to exercise (for example, working out with a friend or trainer; getting a fitness app on your smartphone and adding friends who can support and/or nudge you) may do more for the brain

than exercising alone, and may increase the chances of sticking with an exercise routine.

THE BRASS TACKS: PERSONAL STRATEGIC PLANNING TO ACHIEVE MY EXERCISE GOALS

My current exercise per day / week (circle one):

_____ minutes

Types of exercise I engage in: _____

_____

_____

Where I like to exercise: _____

_____

_____

Time of the day I prefer exercising: _____

_____

_____

Person(s) I like to exercise with: _____

_____

_____

Factors or barriers that get in the way of me exercising more:

_____

_____

_____

Top two things that make it hardest for me to exercise more:

1. _____

_____

2. _____

_____

Strategies that I can use to overcome exercise barrier #1:

_____

_____

_____

Strategies that I can use to overcome exercise barrier #2:

_____

_____

_____

Small steps I can take to exercise (even a little bit more) this week: _____

_____

_____

Small steps I can take to exercise (even a little bit more) this month: _____

_____

_____

Exercise goals I have for myself over the next 3 months:

_____

_____

_____

Exercise goals I have for myself over the next 6 months:

_____

_____

_____

Things I've learned from this chapter that could help me
exercise more: _____

_____

_____

How exercising more is consistent with my current values:

_____

_____

_____

6

Socializing and the Brain: Stay Connected to Improve Your Neural Connections

WHILE NOT A SOCIAL BUTTERFLY BY ANY MEANS, Gene was the type of person who tried to push himself to stay engaged with others. Twice a week, he would meet with a handful of friends for "coffee club" at a local café. Conversations were good (often better than the coffee), and he found it was a stimulating way to start the day. I saw Gene periodically over a few years, and despite having some mild cognitive problems in our initial evaluation, he didn't show increased memory difficulties over time. Multiple factors come into play when we understand why people do or do not show cognitive changes, but in Gene's case, I had a hunch that prioritizing social activity with friends was helping his brain stay healthy. Anecdotally, I've seen the same pattern play out in many socially engaged individuals, and the science seems to reinforce what my colleagues and I have observed. Let's look at some of the details.

THE BACKGROUND SCIENCE

This chapter focuses on the relatively new area of inquiry examining the relationship between social activity and brain and cognitive functioning. Recall that social activity is another part of the "A" (*activity engagement*) referenced by the C.A.P.E. model. But what do we mean by *social activity*? We are fundamentally wired to seek out social interaction, and most of us socialize with others on a regular basis in many different ways. Social encounters include impromptu conversations at the grocery store with a neighbor or friend, brief chats with coworkers between meetings, or catching up with a loved one at the end of the day. Perhaps a family dinner at home or on the town, doing volunteer work, being involved in a community group such as a book or garden club, or attending meetings with colleagues are more common in your life.

There are more ways than ever to socialize: face-to-face interaction, making a phone call, video conferencing with a family member or friend, sending an e-mail, writing a text message, or posting on one of the ever-growing forms of social media. In studies that assess social engagement, the way interactions are quantified for research purposes varies but often involves asking people how often they interact with someone for more than 10 minutes at a time.

So, a quick interaction with a store clerk wouldn't count, but coffee with a friend or a slightly extended phone call would.

We know that socializing with people we care about or find interesting is emotionally rewarding . . . and the reverse is emotionally taxing. In addition, scientists have learned fairly recently that positive social interactions are really good for the brain. **The frequency of our social activity, the size of our social network, and our sense of social support all impact cognitive skills and brain health.** Conversely, social isolation and negative social interactions can be detrimental to the brain. In this chapter, we'll look at what the research says in these areas and how the science can guide our decisions about our social lives.

How Does Being Social Keep Us Healthy?

We can all probably relate to the idea that being connected to and supported by others feels good. Maybe it's our relationship with a partner or spouse, a long-standing connection with an old friend or group of friends, positive family ties, or camaraderie with coworkers. When we have these positive interactions, it does something for us in the moment from an emotional standpoint. It also improves our overall health and affects our basic physiology across the life span. We've known for many years that social support helps us manage stress and improves our cardiovascular health. Indeed, people who feel more supported have lower blood pressure, better endocrine function, and stronger immune systems.

Our *social network size* is closely related to social support, and refers to how many people we have meaningful relationships with and see on a fairly regular basis. The size of our social network is also linked to health, and people with more friends and acquaintances tend to be healthier, live longer, and fight disease better. More generally, when we have enriching connections with others, we experience less stress, manage the stress we encounter better, and soak in positive emotion easier. This, in turn, helps the body operate at higher levels. Conversely, feeling less connected can lead us to make proverbial mountains out of molehills. And having fewer social ties sets up an increased risk of various physical problems like obesity and heart disease.

We're also learning more about the relationship between social connections and the brain. For example, when we have positive interactions with other people, the pleasure centers of the brain light up like a Christmas tree (a familiar metaphor in the neuroimaging community). In contrast, negative encounters tend to stir up brain regions that are active when we experience physical pain. This suggests that social tension and physical discomfort are closely related, particularly in terms of how the brain processes these types of experiences.

How Does Social Activity Help the Brain?

There is growing evidence that the more socially active you are, the healthier your brain will be. Increased social activity is associated with better executive functioning, quicker thinking speed, and improvements in some types of memory. These findings are seen across the life span, although the majority of published research has been conducted with older adults. The brain particularly benefits when we engage in multiple social activities rather than just one; a weekly coffee with a friend is good, but adding in time with a hiking club or a community group is better. So how much socializing is necessary for the brain to get a boost? As we'll see, you don't have to become a gregarious social butterfly to reap the brain-based rewards of socializing.

Multiple studies over the past 15 or so years have shown that being socially active translates into improved health and a better-looking and better-working brain. There is also evidence that being socially active reduces the risk of developing dementia. The most powerful studies follow people over the course of time to see whether staying socially engaged helps the brain. Social engagement is usually determined based on the amount of time people spend with friends, family members, or coworkers. The bottom line is that the more we interact with others, the more likely our brain and cognitive skills will be in good shape.

It remains unclear why social activity is so beneficial for the brain, although when you think about the details of a social interaction, the brain clearly gets a solid workout. You need to listen well and comprehend what the other person is saying, read body language (facial expressions, gestures) to interpret the context and emotion of the message, remember how this conversation might be related to distant or recent experiences, think about a response (or decide between multiple responses), and then respond, all in a very short period of time.

We can also think of the emotional benefits of positive interactions: we feel more connected, less stressed-out, and have a better sense of control over our environment. As we'll discuss in Chapter 10, reducing stress in various forms can really help the brain. Getting a mood boost with social activity might be one of the main reasons why the brain benefits when we get together with others. We have less of the potentially noxious hormone cortisol circulating in our bodies when our mood is brighter, and socializing on a regular basis keeps our immune system firing on all cylinders. In addition, emotional support from others quiets the parts of the brain that light up when we feel threatened and ramps up brain regions that respond when we feel safe.

Being more socially active also seems to help our cognitive skills even when we aren't able to do other brain-boosting activities such as exercise, reading, or crossword puzzles. Studies often look at multiple types of activities and account for (or "control for") one activity while analyzing another. In fact, we see that being social is positive for the brain *above and beyond* other activities such as exercise.

A large study a few years ago found that after considering effects of physical and mental activity, people who were
most socially active showed the least amount of memory,
spatial skill, and processing speed decline over a 5-year
period. *Even a small uptick in socializing was found to reduce
cognitive decline by almost 50%.* This study was also interesting because personality type was accounted for; even people
who were more introverted tended to benefit from being
more social. Other research has found that social activity
can enhance our executive function skills—including working memory and mental flexibility—even if we've already
experienced cognitive decline. Notably, there's also evidence
that being more social makes us feel like our memory is
better, even independent of performance on cognitive tests.

How about the social nature of our job? Some people have
jobs where they need to be social throughout the day; others
may be staring into a computer monitor most of the time.
While the latter is not necessarily problematic (though periodically standing up, walking around, and socializing is generally a good idea), people who have more socially active jobs
are less likely to develop cognitive problems such as dementia
later in life. And when we have more socially contained or
isolated jobs, there's evidence that we can make up for being
less social at work by being more social outside of work.

This brings up another issue: Does it matter if our social
activity is at work, at home, in the community, or something
other than face-to-face? We seem to know much more about
the brain-related effects of how much we socialize (and as

we'll talk about soon, the size of our social network) than about how and where we interact with others. In-person social contact is probably better for the brain than e-mail or texting; phone calls and video conferencing may be helpful for brain health (and for promoting positive emotions) but may not be quite as good as being physically present with a loved one.

Some recent research related to prevention of depression has some relevance here. In one large study with more than 10,000 participants, scientists gauged how often people were in touch with friends or family members face-to-face, by phone, or in writing (which included e-mail). Those who were most socially active, which was quantified as three or more social contacts per week, were the least likely to become depressed. While in-person contact was by far the best way to go (particularly with friends), more frequent e-mail contact with others was better than less contact. Frequency of telephone contact didn't seem to matter as much for one's mood as in-person interactions.

Perhaps a lesson we can learn from this study is that when we can interact with others in person—particularly people we like—we should try to prioritize this over a phone call or e-mail, when possible, for the sake of our mood. We can also bridge this idea to brain health. Considering that there are important links between cognitive and emotional function (and dysfunction, particularly depression), we can probably conclude that the more face-to-face interactions we have, the healthier our brain will be.

Social Networks and the Brain

What about the overall size of our social network? Does that confer additional brain-related benefits? Research has a lot to say about this aspect of socializing too. And the bottom line here is that the more people we have in our broader social clan, the better our brain tends to function. Some of the early knowledge in this area came from the so-called Nun Study, where hundreds of nuns were studied over many years (during life, and after death) to help understand why and how some people age better than others.

As we touched on earlier, one of the most remarkable findings from this study related to the appearance of the nuns' brains on autopsy. While some of their brains looked very similar to those with full-blown dementia, during life, many of these nuns were functioning well day to day. In other words, there was something they were doing to reduce the impact of dementia-related brain changes on their daily cognitive skills. One likely possibility is that the breadth of their social networks (in addition to engagement in mental and physical activities) was preventing them from descending into dementia. As we'll see, more recent research findings point in this very direction.

When researchers determine the size of someone's social network, they often ask how many times one has seen a friend or relative over the past month. So, in a way, the bar is set fairly low for the amount of people one interacts with. Many of us see friends or family members on a daily basis. Hopefully you're in this category, but if you're not, there are reasons to connect with new coworkers or people in the community, or to reinvigorate a relationship with an old friend. Some of the more compelling studies have found that the more people you connect with on a regular or semi-regular basis, the less likely you'll show cognitive decline, and the longer you'll live.

A study from the Rush Alzheimer's Disease Center sought to understand whether a larger social network was linked to fewer cognitive problems in people whom they studied for about 5 years. The scientists found that *people with many social connections were almost 40% less likely to experience cognitive decline* than someone with one primary social tie. This finding, and a related result regarding frequency of social activity, was unchanged after accounting for other things that can affect social connectedness, like marital status, educational level, annual income, and physical and mental activity. Other work has shown that the risk of dementia is quite high in those with few or no consistent social contacts, and that each additional person added to your social network—as long as these relationships are satisfying and supportive—further decreases the risk of cognitive impairment as you age.

Following up on our Nun Study discussion, some of the science has more directly linked social network size to the impact of brain changes on our cognitive skills. A fascinating study tried to determine whether social networks could buffer the effects of pathological changes to the brain. They studied older adults who were healthy at the beginning of the study, and determined the social network sizes of these adults via interviews. They also assessed cognitive skills such as working memory and episodic memory using neuropsychological tests. The study participants were tracked cognitively until they passed away. Then the researchers examined the participants' brains, which they had previously agreed to donate to the study. A noble contribution to say the least.

The key result from the study was groundbreaking: the larger the participants' social networks were during life, the less that brain disease affected their cognitive abilities. In other words, even if the autopsied brains appeared to be from individuals who had Alzheimer's disease, the same people didn't show the cognitive impairment usually found in Alzheimer's while they were alive. Further, this pattern played out across multiple types of memory as well as overall cognitive ability. Research like this has poignantly clarified the importance of our social choices on how the brain works, even in the face of neurodegenerative disease.

It is also important to note that social network size isn't everything; the quality of our social interactions is probably just as meaningful. Some research has found that the more satisfied we are with others in our social networks, the less likely we are to develop dementia. As we'll discuss later, frequent interactions that are negative or even toxic can have significant consequences for brain health.

Social Support and the Brain

Diane saw me for a baseline neuropsychological evaluation after being diagnosed with multiple sclerosis (MS). Her physical and cognitive MS symptoms were relatively mild, and she was able to stay fairly active most days. One of the things she really prioritized was seeing friends and family as often as she could. She had quite the social schedule, sometimes visiting or being visited by two or three different people each day. She laughed and told me, "My social life is great, but it's almost exhausting! Seriously, though, I feel fortunate to have a good group of people who seem to like being with me and who I know I can count on if things go south." In the clinic, I observed that her performance on cognitive testing was stable over the course of 4 years. She showed some mild difficulties with cognitive processing speed—common in MS—but minimal worsening over time. The science indicates that people like Diane tend to have more robust brain skills over the years, at least in part because they feel connected to and supported by others.

Beyond the amount of time we spend socializing, or the size of our network, the sense of support we feel from people we interact with is important too. When we're supported by others, we take solace in knowing there's someone we can count on. More generally, we feel less alone in the universe. So, there are clear emotional benefits to having a social safety net. That said, what does social support do for our brains? Is there something about support from others that impacts our cognitive skills and brain health? Fortunately, and as I saw with Diane, the science clearly indicates that the more supported we feel, the better our brains seem to function.

An early study in this area looked at the effects of social support on cognitive aging in a large sample of older adults. At the beginning of the study, the researchers asked the participants about their social lives, including the level of support they felt from others in their social circle. They also assessed multiple thinking skills, which were considered in a global cognitive performance score. Then, 7 years later, the researchers reexamined the participants' cognition.

The most critical factor in determining whether people showed better brain skills since their earlier testing: *social support*. People who felt more supported by others performed better on multiple cognitive tests; those feeling like they were largely on their own showed evidence of poorer brain health. Importantly, these findings remained meaningful above and beyond other factors including physical activity, physical health, psychological status, and annual income. In other words, feeling that others care for us may be more important for brain health than many other life-impacting issues.

Some of the details from earlier research have recently been fleshed out a bit, particularly regarding which cognitive skills benefit from more social support. While some work has found that more social support is related to better overall cognitive functioning, there are also specific benefits for executive functioning (including working memory and task shifting), processing speed, and spatial skills. Some research has found that our sense of being supported well by others is linked to how effectively we can pay attention, and that feeling less supported can negatively affect our verbal memory over time. And there's evidence that feeling the scales of social reciprocity tipping in our favor—a sense that we're receiving more social support than we're giving to others—is tied to a 50% reduced risk of dementia.

One specific aspect of social support that's been looked at is church attendance. A large study that followed over 3,000 Mexican Americans over about 7 years found that those who attended church services at least once a month showed significantly better cognitive functioning than less frequent churchgoers. Factors such as gender, age, and specific religious affiliation did not significantly alter the findings. Similar findings have been observed in African American and Caucasian adults too. Faith comes in many forms, and regardless of denomination, the social cohesion felt in faith communities appears to have many brain-related benefits.

Some people like volunteering in the community—a noble type of social support that usually pays dividends for all involved. Perhaps it's working a few hours a week at a local food bank or homeless shelter; maybe restocking books at a town library is more your style. Beyond the feel-good nature of volunteering for the volunteer—not to mention the benefits for individuals being served and the community at large—volunteering has a nice side benefit that few know about. Simply put, volunteering helps the brain work better, even in people with cognitive problems.

Taking social research out of the laboratory and into the real world can be particularly powerful. A great example of this strategy was a study that examined whether participating in a volunteer program for elementary school children ("Experience Corps") would affect volunteers' *own* cognitive functioning. The volunteers helped with reading skills, library tasks, and classroom activities across the academic year for 15 hours per week. At the end of the school year, compared to those in a control group who did not volunteer, the people in the study showed much better memory and executive functioning (such as organizational skills and flexible thinking). The researchers also found that people with cognitive problems at the beginning of the study showed significant cognitive improvement. It seems intuitive that serving as a volunteer in an elementary or other school would tax and ultimately grow important skills like organization and mental flexibility; this study has the evidence to prove it.

In similar research looking at brain-related changes (using structural and functional neuroimaging), volunteers in the Experience Corps program showed more activity in some frontal lobe areas and greater overall brain volume as a function of their work. Further, the longer they volunteered, the more their brains changed for the better. The findings were particularly notable for volunteers with the highest risk of cognitive problems. The take-home message from these fascinating studies is that engaging in volunteer activity in the community not only helps those receiving the support; the ones providing the service appear to experience healthier brains too.

Troubling Social Experiences and the Brain

We all have challenging interactions from time to time, some more than others. Hopefully the good or neutral interactions outweigh the bad. It's important to consider these separately, because even if we have enriching experiences with some folks, our negative social encounters can essentially erase the cognitive and health-related benefits of positive ones. **Two general types of social challenges are especially problematic: social conflict and social isolation.**

Experiencing strain or conflict with others is an inevitable part of life. Conflict can be a one-time event, such as a negative interaction with a snarky coffee shop employee, or something more chronic, such as marital tension or a challenging relationship with a boss or coworker. Conflicted and positive interactions can certainly occur on a regular basis with the same person. For example, a good lunchtime conversation with a friend can sour when the topic of paying the bill comes up. It perhaps goes without saying that strain with someone we're close to also hits us harder than a negative interaction with someone we don't know as well. On average, and unfortunately, negative interactions tend to be more powerful and stick with us longer than positive ones. It's much easier to ruminate about an encounter that was troubling than one that lifted our spirits.

What does this have to do with the brain? Well, we know that individuals who consistently have negative interactions are less able to regulate cortisol, a hormone that is linked to stress and illness. Cortisol can also damage the brain, especially when it circulates for extended periods of time (we'll talk more about this in Chapter 10). In a related vein, some research has found that social conflict doesn't just have implications for stress levels; social challenges negatively affect how the brain works.

One study followed middle-aged people over a 10-year period. The researchers found that individuals reporting the most negative relationships showed faster decline in executive functioning (in particular, problem solving and verbal fluency) than people with more positive connections. In other words, "accelerated aging" occurred in those with the worst relationships, particularly regarding some executive skills. Curiously, memory wasn't really affected by negative social interactions, suggesting that conflict preferentially degrades only some cognitive abilities.

Another problematic aspect of our social life is when we experience isolation. Being isolated from others can sometimes be hard to avoid—for example, while traveling for work, during illness, or while raising children—but being chronically isolated nevertheless has broad health consequences. For example, research finds negative effects of social isolation on the immune system and blood pressure throughout life. Believe it or not, the health-oriented effects of isolation are not unlike those related to obesity or smoking, including problems with chronic disease, diabetes, and high cholesterol. Even more alarming: older adults who are socially isolated are significantly more likely to die prematurely than those who are more socially connected.

Feeling lonely can also do a number on brain health. Over the course of a decade, people who report loneliness have been found to show more rapid cognitive decline than others, even after considering other social and health factors. In fact, cognitive skills in lonely people have been found to decline 20% faster than in those who don't report feeling lonely. While depression and loneliness can certainly occur together, loneliness itself affects brain health above and beyond our mood state. In a related vein, those with a limited social network show a significantly increased risk of developing cognitive impairment or full-blown dementia, with one study showing that *particularly socially isolated individuals are at a 60% higher risk of cognitive changes.*

These findings serve as a cautionary tale, reminding us not only of the importance of being socially connected, but also of the perils of reducing our social ties. Knowledge is power, and I hope that our discussion here has clarified the implications of both positive and negative interactions as they relate to brain health.

THE BOTTOM LINE

The importance of social interaction and the brain comes down to these key points:

- Frequent social activity (including with friends, family members, or coworkers) is good for emotional and cognitive health.
- Social interactions that last at least 10 minutes have more powerful brain effects than shorter encounters; more social "doses" of this duration are better for the brain.
- Having a relatively large network of social connections is enriching for the brain and reduces the risk of developing dementia.
- If you don't interact with many people at work, make sure you have plenty of social time at home and with friends.
- Feeling a sense of support from others in your life has important emotional and brain-related benefits.
- If you have physical limitations and can't exercise very much, consistent social activity may make up for less time exercising, particularly in terms of brain health.
- Being socially isolated and lonely is toxic to overall health and, specifically, brain health.
- When possible, avoid people who tend to put you in a negative emotional or psychological space.

- Beyond the benefits to those being served, volunteering in the community is associated with brain-related benefits for the volunteer, including better executive functioning and memory, as well as more brain volume.

THE BRASS TACKS:
PERSONAL STRATEGIC PLANNING
TO INCREASE SOCIAL ACTIVITY

Number of people I can rely on and talk with about challenging issues (consider both family members and friends):

_____

These people include: _____

_____

_____

Types of socializing I engage in: _____

_____

_____

Where I like to be social: _____

_____

_____

Factors that get in the way of me socializing more: _____

_____

_____

Top two things that interfere with me being more social:

1. _____

_____

2. _____

_____

Strategies that I can use to overcome social barrier #1:

_____

_____

_____

Strategies that I can use to overcome social barrier #2:

_____

_____

_____

Small steps I can take to socialize (even a little bit more) this week: _____

_____

_____

Small steps I can take to socialize (even a little bit more) this month: _____

_____

_____

Social goals I have for myself over the next 3 months:

_____

_____

_____

Social goals I have for myself over the next 6 months:

_____

_____

_____

Things I've learned from this chapter that could help me become more socially active: _____

_____

_____

How being more socially active is consistent with my current values: _____

_____

_____

The Benefits of Giving Your Brain a Workout: Mental Activities and Hobbies to Embrace

OVER THE YEARS, I HAVE NOTICED THAT SOME OF my patients who seem to stave off cognitive decline are more intellectually active than others. While they may feel that they're not as mentally acute as they used to be, their ongoing interest in reading, playing a musical instrument, or engaging in other stimulating hobbies seems to keep them above water. Research fundamentally supports these observations from the clinic and more generally. **This chapter will consider the science behind mental activity and its value in promoting brain health.** Here, we'll wrap up our discussion of the "A" (*activity engagement*) component of the C.A.P.E. model, after having previously discussed physical activity and social activity in Chapters 5 and 6, respectively.

The importance of staying mentally stimulated is perhaps the most intuitive aspect of the concept of activity engage-

ment for brain health. It just seems to make sense that someone who regularly reads books or the newspaper, does crossword puzzles, and toils away on complicated projects would have a revved-up brain. We now have a fair amount of studies that support this idea, and we'll get into related details here.

THE BACKGROUND SCIENCE

First off, what activities and hobbies are considered to be mentally stimulating? It would be difficult to summarize *all* possibilities, but some of the more common ones that have been researched include:

- Reading the newspaper, magazines, or books
- Doing crossword puzzles, Sudoku, or jigsaw puzzles
- Learning or playing a musical instrument
- Engaging in artistic activities, such as painting, photography, or crafts
- Taking adult or community education courses
- Going to museums
- Traveling to a new place

One of the most important maxims of mental activity and the brain is this: *be willing to be a beginner again.* Try to not be intimidated by attempting something new; on the contrary, embrace the challenge of taking on a hobby that is unfamiliar or difficult. The brain loves to stretch in this way. And, mental cross-training is a good move too. If you're a big reader, great. You're already helping your brain maintain its integrity and are probably growing new neurons. Even better, add crossword puzzles, regular trips to the museum, or a community course from time to time.

Before continuing, we should return to a concept—*cognitive reserve*—that has been used to partly explain why some people do well later in life while others develop mild cognitive impairment or dementia. As you'll recall, cognitive reserve refers to the idea that certain life experiences have a protective influence on brain aging. One of the most commonly considered aspects of cognitive reserve is how much education someone has attained. Multiple studies have shown that people with more education are less likely to develop problems like dementia; even if they develop dementia, they tend to show cognitive decline later than others. We can refer to this type of cognitive reserve as *passive* reserve, in that an earlier life experience continues to exert an indirect influence years later without further effort on our part.

While this idea is encouraging to those who went to high school, then college, and even beyond college, it doesn't account for ongoing mental stimulation throughout one's life. This is what we refer to as *active* cognitive reserve. That is, continuing to build the brain as the years unfold by staying engaged with intellectually demanding (and ultimately rewarding) pursuits. Importantly, we see that people without a lot of early-life education can nevertheless add to their active cognitive reserve by staying mentally stimulated. And, of course, some people have both passive and active reserve going for them. As I like to say to students in my community brain health course, many of whom are older adults, we can continue to build active reserve into our sixties, seventies, and beyond. Fortunately, research finds that both passive and active reserve promote cognitive health and may delay or prevent dementia.

A promising early study followed more than 1,700 cognitively healthy people over time to see whether engaging in mentally stimulating activities might reduce the chances of developing cognitive impairment. Later in the study, about 200 of these people succumbed to dementia. However, those who were the most mentally active in daily life were much less likely to show significant cognitive problems—38% less likely—even after considering other factors such as heart disease or depression. Another interesting finding was that intellectual activity (like reading, playing cards or games, and attending classes) was more protective against dementia than physical or social activity. The other activities mattered, but mental activity was the most powerful in terms of reducing dementia risk.

Other seminal research—an extension of the classic Nun Study—found that individuals who were moderately active with hobbies such as reading or crossword puzzles had about a 28% reduced risk of Alzheimer's disease. Even better, compared to people who were mentally sedentary, those who were most active were almost twice as likely to avoid this devastating condition. And a review and meta-analysis of many studies in this area concluded that participation in activities that stretched the brain was linked to improved memory, processing speed, and executive functioning skills. More generally, being involved with a hobby of interest is associated with better overall health, including reduced blood pressure, less depression and anxiety, improved ability to cope with stressful events, and lower levels of cortisol (a key stress hormone).

On the other hand, and important to keep in mind: less mental activity has been linked to atrophy of the medial temporal lobe—the home of some of our most crucial memory skills. Engaging in almost anything mentally engaging is doing something positive for the brain, which we'll learn more about next.

Specific Mental Activities That Matter

Most of the research looking at the effects of mental activity on brain health—and reduced risk of dementia—examines a number of different activities together. However, some studies either consider specific activities in isolation or allow us to extrapolate which activities among many seem to matter the most. For example, reading books, newspapers, or magazines has been found to be particularly important in reducing dementia risk. Reading on a regular basis might even have a more protective effect on the brain than the years of education one has attained. This is a particularly important finding given that education is often considered to be the most important component of one's cognitive reserve. While some people are not able to complete as much formal education as they'd like, reading is an accessible way for all to *actively* build cognitive reserve. Other studies have found that reading reduces the risk of developing milder cognitive problems and improves our ability to appreciate others' perspectives (especially as a function of reading fiction). It's safe to say that reading in any form is a very brain-healthy activity.

In my clinic, after discussing neuropsychological evaluation findings, patients will often ask whether crossword puzzles do anything meaningful for brain health. For many years, I didn't have a great answer to give them. Now, I can mention a specific study that supports the powerful brain effects of being a cruciverbalist (fancy term for crossword puzzler).

In the study, about 500 older adults—all without cognitive problems at baseline—were followed over the course of time. One hundred and one of them eventually developed Alzheimer's disease or other forms of dementia. The authors discovered something fascinating about the puzzlers: people who worked on crossword puzzles as little as once per week delayed their memory impairment by 2½ years compared to non-puzzlers. If we can generalize these findings to daily life, it means that doing one crossword puzzle per week might serve a protective effect against dementia as we age. Chalk that up as another inexpensive mental activity that can make a real difference for brain health.

Maybe you like playing cards or checkers? Or doing jigsaw puzzles? One study lumped these activities (and crossword puzzles) together into a "playing games" category in their research. The researchers then tried to determine whether engaging in these sorts of activities had any meaningful effects on the brain. Fortunately, they did: people who played games more often had better working memory, verbal learning and memory, processing speed, mental flexibility, and spatial skills. That's quite a list! Even more intriguing was the finding that playing games was more important than the complexity of one's job in promoting some cognitive abilities. We'll talk about the positive effects of work-related mental demands later in the chapter, but suffice it to say that leisure activities such as playing cards or checkers might be more important for the brain than we've previously believed.

Another study investigated common leisure activities like reading, playing board games, and dancing. The researchers followed a group of older adults for 5+ years and determined whether mentally engaging hobbies had a protective effect against developing dementia. They definitely did. In particular, *people who were most mentally engaged had a 63% lower risk of dementia than those who didn't engage in much mental activity.* Another compelling finding from this study was that every daily increase in cognitive activity—such as reading or playing board games an additional day per week—was linked to a 7% lower risk of cognitive impairment. Let's say you read at night twice per week. Based on this research, reading one or two more nights per week could reduce your dementia risk by an additional 7% to 14%. That's pretty powerful, especially given that you'd be doing something you already like, just slightly more often.

If you happen to play a musical instrument or would like to, your brain has some good news for you: it really likes to be stimulated in this way. Multiple peer-reviewed studies have found that the challenges and joys that come along with creating music are also associated with improvements in a few cognitive abilities. As those of you who play piano, guitar, bass, clarinet, or any other instrument can attest, learning a new piece can take quite a bit of mental effort.

A study from scientists at the University of Southern California looked at pairs of twins to determine whether playing an instrument reduced the likelihood of developing dementia. As with other so-called twin studies, this type of research is particularly interesting because twins have either identical or similar genes and, for those raised together, also experienced similar things growing up. In turn, we can look more precisely at specific factors that might help one twin's brain health and harm or reduce it in the other.

This study looked at twins who were discordant for playing an instrument; that is, one twin played an instrument and the other didn't. The researchers found something startling: the twin who played an instrument was 64% less likely to develop dementia than their non-musical co-twin, even after accounting for how educated and physically active the twins were. Other studies have found that the more musically engaged one is throughout life, the better one's executive functioning, memory, and other skills tend to be during the aging process. The bottom line seems to be that producing music—at any level—has protective effects on the brain for years to come.

Other activities are associated with better brain fitness too. Perhaps you're into photography or one of the many forms of crafting—there's evidence that engaging in these types of activities can positively impact cognitive skills. One study trained people in digital photography techniques, quilting, or both. The training was fairly intense. The participants were asked to work on their new hobby for 15 hours per week for 3 months straight, so they really dove in. At the end of the study, those who were trained in photography showed significantly better memory compared to their baseline. The new quilters improved almost as much, and people who learned both hobbies also showed memory gains. When you consider what goes into acquiring new skills, it makes sense that these study participants would remember what they were learning, but even more impressive was the general memory improvement.

Variety and Novelty of Activities

We've been discussing the value of specific activities, but what about mental cross-training? Is there something positive about engaging in a few different hobbies that stretch the brain? A study from researchers at Johns Hopkins sought to answer these questions. They asked a large group of older women about the activities they participated in, including how cognitively demanding the activities were. So, doing crossword puzzles or reading were considered to be pretty good workouts for the brain, whereas watching TV wasn't.

Regardless of how mentally intense the activities were, the wider the variety of activities, the more benefits these women reaped. And it really was about *variety*: this mattered more than the *frequency* or *intensity* of the activity. Even the subtitle of their academic article emphasized this point ("variety may be the spice of life"). If you're thinking about adding something to your mental mix, keep this statistic in mind too: each additional brain-bending activity reduced the risk of memory problems and global cognitive impairment by an additional 8% to 11%. Incidentally, these researchers found something similar for exercise: a more varied regimen of physical activity is especially protective against dementia. There seems to be something important to the brain about mixing it up when it comes to activity engagement, particularly regarding hobbies with mental and physical demands.

Another way to consider the issue of variety of mental activities is assessing *novelty seeking*. In other words, does it matter if we try to develop new skills, learn about new topics, or take on a new hobby? There seems to be evidence, as we discussed earlier, that novelty is really good for the brain. We also know that novelty is the frontal lobes' specialty, so it would seem that keeping the frontal cortex busy with fresh activities is a worthy goal.

One study found that over time, people who regularly sought out novel and mentally stimulating activities had a much lower risk of developing dementia. Other research from some of the same scientists found that reducing the time one spends on intellectual hobbies from young adulthood to middle age increases the risk of Alzheimer's disease. Fortunately, the opposite also holds true: people who became increasingly mentally active as they got older showed reduced dementia risk.

As we might expect, people who are involved not only in a variety of mental activities, but a broader variety of activities including exercise and social engagement, are generally better off. This relates to our discussion in Chapter 5 about *dose–response relationships* vis-à-vis brain health; increases in the amount of time spent on activities tend to result in better brain functioning. Research from a few years ago found that while participating in one type of activity was helpful, an increased "dose" of two or more activities reduced the risk of dementia significantly.

In terms of how much time you should engage in mentally stimulating hobbies for better brain health, there seems to be evidence that spending at least an hour per day is particularly effective at lowering the risk of cognitive problems down the road. A study with older adults assessed how much time people did things such as read books or newspapers, play board games, complete crossword puzzles, play musical instruments, or work on crafts. People who were involved with these types of leisure activities for at least an hour a day had a significantly lower risk of dementia compared to those engaging for fewer than 30 minutes per day. As with other research we've discussed, a wider variety of hobbies also had a protective effect against dementia.

Start Now . . . Midlife Mental Activity Matters

I'd like to mention a related point that we considered earlier in the book: *midlife activity plays a vitally important role in late-life cognitive status.* As with physical and social engagement in our forties and fifties, mentally stimulating activity in midlife reduces the chances of developing mild cognitive impairment or dementia down the road. If you're reading this book and you're roughly aged 40 to 60, you're doing the right thing by staying mentally stimulated. You probably realize this intuitively, but science definitely backs up this hunch.

If you're in your forties, one study might motivate you to keep your brain firing right now. The study assessed mental activity in midlife in male twins, where one twin later developed dementia and the other remained cognitively healthy. The twin pairs were tracked over time, and about 30 years later, it turned out that the twins with dementia had been much less cognitively active in midlife. Curiously, the activities at midlife that seemed to be most protective against dementia were going out to the movies, attending a theatrical event, or seeing live music. I suspect that the social and intellectual components of these activities were particularly helpful. So, if you have the opportunity to catch an upcoming movie or concert, and you need some justification to do so, just remember that you might be helping your brain in ways that will pay off years from now.

If you're in your fifties, the pattern seems to be about the same. A large study followed people for about 20 years who began the research in their late fifties. At the beginning of the study, participants were interviewed and asked about a wide variety of lifestyle activities. The goal was to clarify what types of activities—including mentally stimulating ones—were linked to skills such as attention and memory many years later. The findings indicated that middle-aged people who were more frequently engaged mentally (reading books, playing a musical instrument, doing other hobbies) and politically (participating at a political demonstration, writing an article or letter to the editor) had better cognitive skills decades later. The latter result was particularly intriguing; while we live in politically tumultuous times, it's important to note that being involved in politics at some level appears to have some brain-related benefits.

For those of us in the workforce, another area to consider in midlife is the stimulating nature of our job. Given how much time we spend at work, it only makes sense that what we do at work should matter from a brain-based standpoint, right? In fact, the science supports this idea. A study from a few years ago looked at the complexity of one's job in three domains: data, people, or things. What the research-ers found was that a more complex job protected against atrophy of the entire brain, and specifically against atrophy of the memory-critical hippocampus. Of particular interest, though, was the finding that complexity related to people—that is, the experience of workers in managerial roles—was most protective against worrisome brain changes.

On the other hand, if you're in a job that doesn't really stimulate you mentally, there's hope from a cognitive stand-point. Some research has found that people can in a sense make up for a cognitively dull job by staying engaged outside of work. In fact, being a reader, doing hobbies, and going to the movies or the theater is associated with better brain skills in the future *independent* of how complex one's job is or has been. Also note that some brain-boosting mental tasks we've discussed involve social activity: a great one-two punch.

Brain-Training Games

As a side note of sorts, I wanted to mention a topic that I'm frequently asked about: do computerized "brain-training" games help our cognitive skills or even prevent dementia? These apps and programs are very popular, but we need to consider what the science has to say. The popularity of an idea isn't necessarily a good indicator of its validity, so it's important to understand whether research backs up the claims that companies with these products sometimes make regarding brain health.

Take a step back for a moment, and consider skills you have that took a while to develop. Examples might include driving, cooking certain dishes, playing card games, or completing work-related tasks. You needed some time to figure out how to do these things, but eventually you got better, perhaps even mastered them. But ask yourself a question: Did improvement on a specific task (like driving or cooking) generalize to other tasks? If you developed better eye–hand coordination when you learned to drive, did you find that other unrelated tasks that involved similar skills improved too? Usually this isn't the way things pan out.

The same issue has been investigated with brain-training games: whether using them is linked to better cognitive skills in daily life. The general scientific consensus at this point seems to be that they're not. As with driving or cooking, the more you do it, the better you get. But that doesn't mean that you'll necessarily get better at other activities that involve similar demands.

In a comprehensive review of the science to date, scientists examined a wide variety of individual brain-training studies (over 130 separate studies). They found that people get better at games they're introduced to—usually quite a bit better—but the skills that improve on specific games don't seem to boost cognitive performance in daily life. A recent meta-analysis that examined more than 300 studies in this area essentially found the same thing.

What's also interesting is that when people are led to believe that video-game training will improve their cognition, it just might. One study recruited people by using two types of flyers. One suggestive flyer indicated that the study involved brain training, and it cited research that showed intellectual gains due to working memory training. The other flyer was bland and generic, and it mentioned that people participating in the study could earn up to five student credits. Not terribly exciting, right?

It turns out that the people who joined the study thinking they would experience improvement (based on the flyer they read) did better than the other group on an intelligence test after just 1 hour of training. The researchers argued that this group didn't improve in a way that would last from there on out, but rather showed rapid gains during the study because they were led to believe that they would. This is what is referred to as a placebo effect or expectancy effect; the participants in the study improved because they expected to, or perhaps tried harder than people enrolling just for course credits. Curiously, in the description of their research findings, the authors mentioned that other studies in this area have used similarly suggestive strategies to recruit participants. The scientists concluded that an intervention that purports to do something positive for the brain might succeed at some level, but that at least some of the effect—and perhaps most if not all of the effect—may be related to one's expectations rather than the "treatment" itself.

So, if you're interested in getting better at certain types of games, brain training might be for you. And some scientists do see the potential for brain games to augment our cognitive skills. But if you're more interested in what the majority of the science says—that these products don't seem to show meaningful effects in daily life, at least not yet—you might want to focus on other ways to stimulate your mind.

THE BOTTOM LINE

Here are some key takeaways related to mental activity and the brain:

- Taking on a hobby that is novel and challenging is particularly good for the brain.
- Participating in hobbies and other mentally stimulating activities in midlife appears to have a strong protective effect on the brain that lasts for decades and is associated with a reduced risk of dementia.
- Specific activities such as reading, doing crossword puzzles, playing games, photography, and playing a musical instrument are all associated with better cognitive health.
- Engaging in a variety of different mentally stimulating activities might be better than frequently doing any one activity: think "mental cross-training."
- Any hobby participation is positive, but an hour or more per day has a particularly powerful and protective effect on the brain.
- Working in a complex and stimulating job, especially if you're managing others, has brain-enhancing benefits.

- If you're in a job that isn't very stimulating, you can make up for this cognitively by pursuing mentally engaging hobbies.
- Research to date indicates that improvement on computerized brain-training games does not seem to result in cognitive gains in daily life.

THE BRASS TACKS: PERSONAL STRATEGIC PLANNING TO INCREASE MENTAL ACTIVITY

Mentally stimulating activities or hobbies I engage in:

_____

_____

_____

Amount of time I spend per day/per week engaging in these activities: _____

_____

Time of the day I prefer engaging in the above activity or activities: _____

_____

Factors that get in the way of me engaging in more mental activity: _____

_____

_____

Top two things that make it hardest for me to engage in mental activities more:

1. _____

_____

2. _____

_____

Strategies that I can use to overcome mental activity barrier #1:

_____

_____

_____

Strategies that I can use to overcome mental activity barrier #2:

_____

_____

_____

Mental activities or hobbies I'd like to engage in more:

_____

_____

_____

Small steps I can take to engage in a mental activity (even a little bit more) this week: _____

_____

_____

Small steps I can take to engage in a mental activity (even a little bit more) this month: _____

_____

_____

Mental activity goals I have for myself over the next 3 months: _____

_____

_____

Mental activity goals I have for myself over the next 6 months: _____

_____

_____

Things I've learned from this chapter that could help me become more mentally active: _____

_____

_____

How being more mentally active is consistent with my current values: _____

_____

_____

PART III

Other Ways to Potentially Prevent Cognitive Problems

8

Your Brain Is What You Eat: Nutrition and Cognition

FAD DIETS HAVE COME AND GONE FOR DECADES, and more are certainly on the horizon. People often choose a diet hoping to lose weight. Perhaps they've heard about a trendy diet that offers a quick weight-loss plan before summer to look better in a swimsuit. Or they have a friend who has tried a dietary plan that has worked well for him or her. **While there are many reasons to modify one's diet, note that this chapter is focused on the importance of dietary choices from a brain health perspective.** Our discussion and the related changes you may decide to make could lead to weight loss, but the main goal here is to consider the connections between what we eat and how our brain works.

An important caveat: I am not a nutritionist, and you should always consult with a physician, nutritionist, or related professional when considering a dietary change. That being said, there is a fairly large body of research devoted to investigating brain-healthy dietary styles. Much of the science has examined dietary choices that reduce the risk of cognitive decline or dementia in older adults, although some research has looked at nutrition in younger groups too, particularly in midlife. In a related vein, recent research has found that losing weight doesn't necessarily impact overall mortality, or risk of premature death. In fact, the science indicates that one can be overweight and still be fairly healthy, as long as one's physical fitness level is relatively high.

Another point to emphasize is that there is no single food, vitamin, or nutritional supplement that will quickly or magically transform your brain. If you read something about such a claim, you can probably debunk it immediately. Nutritional factors gradually affect our cognitive skills over time and can ultimately have powerful effects on how the brain operates. But there simply isn't a "better brain health in 7 days" diet—or 14 days, or 30 days, or another brief time frame—that stands up to scientific scrutiny. Please keep this in mind as we discuss the scientific evidence related to dietary patterns and some specific nutrients and foods.

Given that eating well plays an important role in maintaining cognitive functioning and potentially preventing brain-related problems, this chapter falls into the "P," or *prevention*, category in our now-familiar C.A.P.E. model. Hungry for more information? (Sorry, couldn't resist that one.) Let's see what the science says about nutrition and the brain.

THE BACKGROUND SCIENCE

People I work with sometimes ask: Does what I eat affect my brain? Are there any foods I should eat more than others? I've heard I should eat a lot of blueberries—is that true? **A number of studies have addressed these and related questions, and we can now provide evidence-based perspectives on what foods are good for the brain and what foods we should try to avoid or cut back on.**

In 2017, AARP conducted a study that clarified dietary habits in a large and ethnically diverse group of middle-aged and older Americans (age 40+). The study participants were asked to describe their food consumption related to five basic food groups—fruits, vegetables, protein, dairy, and grains—and also to rate their well-being and perceived brain health. Note that while brain health in this study was based on subjective impressions rather than cognitive test scores, the research we'll review later does examine cognitive performance in the context of nutrition.

The positive findings: People who eat the USDA-recommended amount of fruits (1.5 to 2 cups per day) and vegetables (2 to 3 cups per day) reported higher well-being and better brain functioning. And there was a dose–response effect too. The more fruits and veggies, the better people reported their brain health to be. Also, those who ate fish but not red meat in a typical week reported having stronger cognitive skills, and the same pattern emerged for people who usually ate nuts. Cooking with olive oil, canola oil, or grapeseed oil was more linked to perceived brain health than vegetable oil. Incidentally, people who eat a fair amount of fish, nuts, and olive oil are eating along the lines of the Mediterranean-style diet, which we'll review shortly.

The sobering findings: A remarkably low 1% of study participants met recommended nutritional standards in all five food groups. And 34% of people said they didn't eat the recommended amount of food in *any* food group. Those who have sugary desserts or drinks and prepared foods at least weekly were less likely to rate their brain health as "excellent" or "very good." Curiously, even though most people didn't follow nutritional standards very well, almost 90% said they would eat better if they knew it would lead to better brain and heart health. Over half said they would potentially change their diet if advised to do so by their doctor.

As with barriers to exercise, there are various reasons why people such as those in the AARP study find it difficult to eat healthy foods. Some of the common barriers include high cost, concerns that more nutritious foods don't taste as good, and limited access to healthy foods. Even personally identifying as "not being a healthy-foods type" negatively affects dietary choices. On the other hand, factors such as family traditions, medical advice, and perceived health benefits tend to motivate people to eat healthier. As we consider the science behind dietary styles and specific foods known to be good for brain health, we also need to remember that there are important social and cultural factors that also determine what we do and don't eat.

Mediterranean and Related Dietary Styles

In terms of a dietary style with solid scientific evidence related to promoting brain health, nothing comes closer than the Mediterranean diet. You may have heard about this style of eating but are unclear what it refers to; essentially, the name references dietary tendencies among people who live in the Mediterranean region (think Italy, Greece, France, Spain, and the Middle East). The diet is mostly plant-based and consists of lots of fruits and vegetables, beans, nuts, and whole grains (Figure 8.1). Olive oil is emphasized, particularly for cooking. Moderate amounts of fish and poultry are included. A little red wine is generally considered part of the "package" too. Foods that are de-emphasized include red meat, high-fat dairy products, and processed items (as I've heard at least one nutritionist say, "foods that your great grandmother wouldn't recognize"). Also included in the broader diet are lifestyle choices, such as moderate physical activity, social engagement, and adequate daily rest and nightly sleep. Let's look at the science that connects the Mediterranean diet (often referred to by researchers as the "MeDi") with brain function.

A wide variety of nutritional studies reveal the same thing: the MeDi plays a protective role against mild or more troubling cognitive problems. The findings differ slightly across the science, but the majority of research shows a significantly reduced risk of mild cognitive impairment (MCI) or Alzheimer's disease—*about a 20% to 40% reduced risk*—in

Foods to Emphasize:
Fruits   Vegetables   Olive Oil   Legumes (beans, lentils, peanuts, chick peas)   Nuts/Seeds (walnuts, almonds, pistachios) Cereals/Bread/Pasta/Rice/Couscous (preferably whole grain) Herbs/Spices/Garlic/Onions (for seasoning) 6 to 8 Glasses of Water per Day

Low to Moderate Amounts of:
Fish   White Meat (chicken/turkey)   Eggs Yogurt and Cheese (preferably low fat) Red Wine (during meals, if desired)

Avoid or Minimize:
Red Meat   Processed Meat   Other Processed Foods High-Fat Dairy Products   Sugary Foods   Soda Drinks

FIGURE 8.1 Components of the Mediterranean Diet

those who consistently eat lots of MeDi foods like fish, olive oil, fruits, and vegetables. Fundamentally, it seems that the more you eat this way, the more brain protection you have. There is also less risk of converting from MCI to dementia in those who maintain this diet over time. Considering that many people diagnosed with MCI eventually develop Alzheimer's disease, lifestyle strategies that potentially prevent this conversion to dementia are desperately needed. As another key benefit, there's a lower risk of stroke and depression in those who follow a Mediterranean-style diet.

One study a few years ago evaluated the diets of over 2,000 people to see whether increased adherence to the

MeDi translated into a lower risk of cognitive problems. The subjects were rated on a 0 to 9 scale to determine how well they stuck to a Mediterranean-style diet ("0" meant essentially no meaningful commitment to the MeDi; "9" meant strong commitment). Over a 4-year period, people who were moderately committed to the diet (a score of 4 or 5 on their MeDi scale) had a 20% reduced risk of dementia. Those who really adhered to the MeDi (a score of 6 to 9) were—remarkably—40% less likely to develop Alzheimer's disease compared to those who were not interested in this diet. So, a higher "dose" of the MeDi was much more protective for the brain than a lower one.

This dose–response effect resembles what we've discussed in earlier chapters: the more people engage in a brain-healthy activity or lifestyle choice, the lower the chance of having significant cognitive problems. Notably, the study also found that eating specific foods within the MeDi—like fruits, fish, or legumes—was less powerful in reducing one's risk of dementia than committing to the entire diet. We'll discuss some of the science on specific foods later, but suffice it to say that broader dietary patterns seem to matter more than individual foods in ramping up brain health.

For people who struggle to exercise consistently, or who are simply unable to exercise much due to physical limitations, there's a MeDi study that offers hope from a brain health perspective. A large group of older adults was asked how much they exercised and how much they adhered to the MeDi. While people who exercised more than others had a much lower chance of developing Alzheimer's disease—consistent with our earlier discussion of the exercise–brain relationship—diet mattered too. Those who followed the MeDi particularly well over the course of about 5 years had a significantly reduced risk of Alzheimer's disease, even if they were relatively sedentary. In other words, eating in a brain-healthy way had a protective effect on the brain *independent* of physical activity levels.

Why is the MeDi so good for the brain? It seems that this nutritional regimen affects the brain on a number of levels. On a microscopic, molecular level, it's rich in antioxidants and anti-inflammatory components that reduce the negative effects of what is called *oxidative stress*—too many potentially toxic free-radical molecules—on the brain. The diet may also have antithrombotic and antiatherogenic features, which is a fancy way of saying that it reduces the risk of strokes and clogged arteries. Flavonoids and polyunsaturated fatty acids (such as omega-3 fatty acids) are abundant in this diet too; we'll discuss these more later.

When we consider the effects of the MeDi on brain structure and volume, we see how this dietary style promotes brain health on a larger scale. All else being equal, more brain volume equates to a better working brain. People adhering to the MeDi have denser brain matter in multiple regions—including in the frontal and temporal lobes—and show reduced shrinkage or atrophy of the brain over time. Less dietary intake of red meat and dairy products, and more fish consumption—along the lines of the MeDi—is associated with higher brain volume. People eating the MeDi also have brain regions showing better *structural connectivity*, or being more intimately linked. The saying "you are what you eat" really applies here, particularly in terms of the brain.

While we've reviewed compelling evidence that supports adhering to a Mediterranean-style diet, diets with similar features have also been studied. One such diet is the DASH diet, which stands for Dietary Approaches to Stop Hypertension. The primary difference between the DASH and MeDi diets is that the DASH diet emphasizes foods with low sodium and low saturated fat; other foods are about the same. While this dietary style was originally designed to prevent or reduce high blood pressure, it has some brain-related benefits too. Among the few studies in this area, people eating in a DASH style have been found to show better overall cognitive functioning and quicker thinking speed. They also have a reduced risk of developing Alzheimer's disease. The research has looked at people on the DASH diet over the course of anywhere from 4 months to 11 years, so it appears that the cognitive benefits can really persist over time.

Another study created what was termed a *healthy eating index*. People aged 55 and older were given higher scores when they ate more fruits, vegetables, whole grains, soy protein, and fish. This was an impressive study: over 27,000 people across 40 countries were followed for 4 to 5 years. Studying that many people, especially over multiple years, is no small task! Another interesting detail of note is that study participants had some sort of medical problem, like diabetes, heart disease, or neurologic disease. Many studies have very healthy subjects that are free of any medical issues, and because this one doesn't fall into that category, it may apply more to the average person with a condition that is being monitored or treated medically.

While some of the participants showed cognitive decline during the study, those who maintained a particularly healthy diet—such as eating lots of fruits, veggies, and whole grains—had a *24% reduced risk of showing cognitive decline.* There were particular benefits of this diet for concentration ability. The researchers also found that people eating in this way who exercised at least twice per week had an even lower risk of cognitive problems. As we've seen in other studies, healthy lifestyle choices in one area (say, physical activity) are good for the brain; healthy choices in multiple areas are even better.

An additional dietary style that is associated with cognitive health is what researchers have called a *prudent diet.* One study used statistical techniques to determine who preferred one of two general dietary tendencies. The components of the prudent diet included vegetables, fruit, legumes (like peas, beans, lentils, and peanuts), rice, pasta, whole grains, water, fish, and poultry. The other dietary category was the *Western diet,* a catch-all term for a diet with red meat, potatoes, pastries, soda, beer, sugar, refined grains, and high-fat dairy products. The scientists then determined how much people leaned toward either or both of these styles of eating.

Over the course of about 6 years, the people who

adhered most to the prudent diet showed the least decline on a cognitive measure that looked at things like concentration, memory, language, and spatial skills. In contrast, people who loved steaks and potatoes—the Western diet fans—had the most cognitive decline. To be fair, many people enjoy hamburgers *and* fish. One night's dinner might be salmon and pasta; the next, a meat-lover's pizza. Fortunately, the researchers found something encouraging for those with a more diverse palate: people eating a Western diet showed much less cognitive decline over time if they regularly made healthy, "prudent" nutritional choices too. While the prudent diet was the best way to go, it could also serve to reduce the brain health risks of the Western diet for those who prefer both dietary styles.

Why is the Western diet bad for the brain? Some research suggests that this dietary style, which is high in saturated fat and refined sugar, has particularly negative effects on the brain's frontal cortex and hippocampus. It turns out that at the molecular level, these areas are sensitive to diets with poor nutritional content, particularly regarding reduced levels of brain-derived neurotrophic factor, or BDNF. (We discussed BDNF in the chapter on exercise and the brain, and how BDNF plays a critically important role in helping the brain grow new neurons and nurture existing ones.) Less BDNF is also linked to inflammation in the brain, which can potentially lead to conditions such as Alzheimer's disease. In addition, oxidative stress occurs in diets with more fat and fewer antioxidants—essentially the opposite of what we see in the MeDi and other non-Western diets. Oxidative stress, in turn, can lead to negative brain changes, including less volume in the frontal lobes.

All told, it seems that a dietary style that de-emphasizes saturated fat and refined sugar seems to be the best way to go. While this makes sense from a broader health perspective, it's a sensible way to promote brain health too.

Specific Foods That Can Boost Brain Health

So far, we've been discussing brain-friendly diets that involve a variety of different foods. **What about specific foods we should be eating more frequently for their cognitive perks?** In general, a broad approach to dietary choices seems to be ideal: it's better to eat a Mediterranean-style diet, with its collective benefits, than to focus on one specific food. However, there are some foods that are particularly advantageous for the brain according to neuroscience research.

While you probably weren't that interested in the childhood nudging you may have gotten about fruits and vegetables, such advice is actually pretty relevant for brain health. One study from a few years ago assessed fruit and vegetable consumption in a large sample of older women. Eating a lot or a little fruit, particularly citrus fruit, didn't seem to matter much for brain health. But the women who ate more cruciferous or green leafy vegetables—like broccoli, kale, cauliflower, and spinach—showed memory and general cognitive decline that was 1 to 2 years slower than in people who ate significantly fewer vegetables. The science presents a convincing case that mom was right all along.

Another study found something similar: consuming leafy vegetables was linked to slower cognitive decline over the course of 6 years. For people who ate at least two servings of veggies per day, it was like they were 5 years younger from a cognitive standpoint. Pretty impressive to say the least: a salad and a side of broccoli each day could pack quite a punch against cognitive problems later in life.

Some recent nutritional research has further clarified the connection between vegetables and cognition. Scientists looked at the frequency of eating green leafy vegetables in a large group of middle-aged and older adults, and how this dietary choice related to cognitive health over about 5 years. The results were compelling: eating 1 to 2 daily servings of veggies was associated with significantly fewer cognitive changes over time, *comparable to being 11 years younger* than those who didn't eat many—if any—vegetables. Specific nutrients in vegetables that were particularly important included lutein, folate, and phylloquinone (also known as vitamin K1). While these aren't familiar to most people outside of a doctor's or nutritionist's office, they may become so in the future given their emerging brain-related benefits.

We now know that vegetables are important both for the body in general and the brain in particular. Large surveys indicate, however, that most people don't eat vegetables consistently. Only about 10% of people have a serving of vegetables each day—which the Centers for Disease Control and Prevention defines as 2 to 3 cups. Considering the research we've discussed, we can speculate that if more people simply had a spinach or kale salad each day, we might see the rates of some cognitive disorders (like Alzheimer's disease) decline, perhaps significantly.

Even though the existing science suggests that vegetables have the brain health advantage over fruits, there is some evidence that one type of fruit stands out: *berries*. Berries are chock-full of flavonoids, which have been found to boost brain health in multiple studies using laboratory animals. Flavonoids are thought to be particularly important for the brain given their antioxidant properties and ability to reduce inflammation. Human research has shown that people who eat more berries show less cognitive decline, better working memory, and increased blood flow in multiple brain regions. They also tend to report fewer problems with executive functioning skills in daily life.

The largest study to date looking at blueberries and cognition enrolled more than 16,000 older women. As with other research we've discussed, the bigger the study sample, the more likely the findings are to be accurate and of importance. The women were asked how often they consumed blueberries, strawberries, other fruits, and tea. After accounting for other factors such as participant age, income, education level, and physical activity, the people who ate the most blueberries and strawberries showed significant delays in memory and other cognitive decline—

delays of up to 2½ years—compared to peers who were less interested in berries. Keep in mind that the berry fans weren't necessarily eating them all the time; the high "berry intake" group in the study was eating at least 1 to 2 servings per week (about 3 to 4 cups). We're not talking grizzly bear levels of berry munching, just keeping the intake slow and steady.

Along these lines, a relatively new dietary style builds on the Mediterranean diet and emphasizes berry and green leafy vegetable intake. So far, it's shown impressive results regarding brain health. It's called the MIND diet—the Mediterranean DASH Intervention for Neurodegenerative Delay—and it essentially adds the benefits of the DASH diet to the MeDi. The MIND diet has been found to have some real advantages: it's been linked to stronger verbal memory and reduced risk of Alzheimer's disease in middle-aged and older adults. It can also slow the process of cognitive aging; people that really abide by this diet have cognitive skills over 7 years younger than their chronological age.

We discussed the Mediterranean diet earlier and mentioned the inclusion of fish in the context of the broader diet. A few studies have specifically looked at fish consumption in isolation. In one, researchers asked a group of older adults how much fish they ate, and then followed these people for about 8 years. The participants in the study were lumped into two groups: those who ate fish one to four times per week, and those who ate less. Unfortunately, if you're a (fried) fish-n-chips fan, you would have been disqualified from this one. Fish consumption had to be of the baked or broiled variety.

Findings were very positive for fish lovers. People who consumed at least a serving of fish per week at the beginning of the study showed more brain mass in multiple regions years later. These areas included the memory-critical hippocampus and a region of the frontal lobes called the orbitofrontal cortex. The results were the same even after accounting for physical activity, reflecting a brain-nourishing benefit to eating fish that went above and beyond the effects of another important lifestyle activity. It's also important to note that the findings could not be chalked up solely to the benefits of omega-3 fatty acids found in fish, as the authors took this factor into account in their analyses.

Other studies indicate that the more baked or broiled fish you eat, the less likely you are to experience subtle or more significant strokes. On the other hand, eating fried fish increases the chances of neurological problems like stroke, and essentially erases the brain-related benefits of eating fish that isn't fried. There just seems to be something about eating non-fried fish that's really good for the brain (and the body). More generally, these results mirror those from earlier chapters: healthy lifestyle choices have a strong impact on brain health.

Other Nutritional Factors Linked to Brain Health

While fish consumption seems important in and of itself, the omega-3 polyunsaturated fatty acids (PUFAs) found in fish and in other products, such as nuts, are also really good for the brain (and the heart and eyes too). PUFAs do many things to promote brain health, such as supporting the functioning of neurons and keeping BDNF and other neurotrophins at normal levels. They also play an important anti-inflammatory role throughout the body and in the brain.

We can't really produce PUFAs ourselves, so it's important that we eat foods with these brain-building components. Two PUFAs in particular—eicosapentaenoic acid (EPA) and docosahexaenoic acid (DHA)—seem especially critical for helping the brain operate at its highest level. These are also referred to as "marine" PUFAs because they are mainly found in fish such as salmon, mackerel, sardines, and tuna. Another one, alpha-linolenic acid (ALA), helps the body synthesize very small amounts of EPA and DHA, though at low enough levels that we really need to get all of these PUFAs from our diet. ALA is found in plants and nuts like walnuts, flax seeds, and soybeans.

More specifically, higher PUFA levels in the body are associated with more brain volume in multiple regions important for memory and executive functioning, such as the hippocampus and cingulate cortex. One study found that higher levels of one of the marine PUFAs, DHA, was associated with a 47% lower risk of any type of dementia. In the same study, where people were followed for about 9 years, eating fish at least three times per week afforded people a 50% reduced risk of Alzheimer's disease compared to those eating less fish. Beyond concerns about dementia, *midlife DHA levels are correlated with better mental flexibility, reasoning, working memory, and word knowledge.* Pretty impressive! This is another example of the importance of keeping our brains healthy and stimulated in midlife (in this case through nutrition), given the potential dividends many years down the road.

While dietary PUFAs are known to be linked to brain wellness, a more controversial position relates to the benefits of taking PUFA supplements. Depending on which doctor or nutritionist you talk to, some recommend supplements and others don't. This is why it's important to consider what the science actually says to inform one's approach to nutrition (and to taking supplements).

Comprehensive reviews and meta-analyses of existing PUFA studies have mostly concluded that PUFA supplementation doesn't reduce the risk of dementia or enhance cognitive health. And a recent yearlong randomized clinical trial comparing PUFAs and placebo pills in older adults found the same thing: no apparent benefit for individuals with mild or no cognitive problems. PUFAs also do not seem to help individuals who have been diagnosed with dementia. While a few studies have found mild cognitive benefits from taking PUFA supplements, most research hasn't. This is also the case regarding cardiovascular health: PUFA supplements don't seem to be associated with a lower risk of heart disease or heart attacks. **The bottom line is that it's better to get brain-healthy nutrients *through one's diet* rather than through supplements.**

Many of my patients have asked about the role of antioxidant compounds on brain health. The ones that have been investigated the most include vitamins C and E and beta-carotene. Large individual studies and reviews of smaller studies have generally not found a consistent benefit for the brain from these antioxidants, although a few positive findings have been observed for vitamin C. The studies in this area have had some problems, such as measuring cognitive skills using simple screening measures rather than more sophisticated neuropsychological tests. So, the evidence isn't very compelling at this point to take antioxidants primarily for the purpose of improving brain function.

You may have heard online or in the news about the benefits of curcumin on the brain. This is a pigment that comes from the turmeric plant and is most often found in curry. While it has been used for many years in Indian medicine, only recently has curcumin been investigated for its potential effects on brain structure and function. There have been some encouraging findings linking curcumin to improved neurological health in animal research, but only a few small studies have been conducted in humans. At this point, the jury's still out on the possible benefits of curcumin for the human brain and our cognitive skills. That said, if you're a curry fan, there's certainly no need to hesitate, and it might just do good things for your taste buds *and* your brain.

What about other over-the-counter supplements? A recent study that reviewed about 40 individual studies of compounds like ginkgo biloba and B vitamins wasn't encouraging. The general finding was that there was either no or weak evidence supporting the role of supplements in preventing cognitive decline. In turn, the scientists concluded that there wasn't justification to recommend these or other supplements to promote brain health. A meta-analysis examining the effects of ginkgo biloba on dementia did find some benefits compared to placebo pills, although again, this was in people with significant cognitive impairment, not the average person.

All told, there simply isn't convincing evidence that currently available supplements do anything meaningful for the brain. Fortunately, as we've discussed throughout the book thus far, there are plenty of other things we know of that are effective at promoting brain health.

THE BOTTOM LINE

In summary, here are a few particularly critical points from our chapter on brain health and nutrition:

- A Mediterranean-style diet seems to be the best nutritional choice for promoting brain health based on a number of studies.
- A Western diet, with its emphasis on red meat, potatoes, and high-fat dairy products, is associated with weaker cognitive functioning.
- Combining a Mediterranean-style or prudent diet with a Western diet reduces the risk of cognitive decline.
- A diet containing more fish than red meat is associated with better brain health.
- Across studies, foods that can enhance cognitive skills include fish, nuts, olive oil, fruit, and vegetables.
- Leafy green vegetables (spinach) and cruciferous vegetables (broccoli, kale, cauliflower) have been linked to slower cognitive decline during the aging process.
- Berries—particularly blueberries and strawberries—have been found in some studies to be protective against memory and general cognitive decline.
- Omega-3 fatty acids, ingested through one's diet rather than as supplements, have been associated with better cognitive functioning, larger brain volume, and reduced risk of dementia.
- No available over-the-counter nutritional supplements have consistently been found to improve cognitive skills.

THE BRASS TACKS:
PERSONAL STRATEGIC PLANNING
TO ACHIEVE MY DIETARY GOALS

My current diet generally consists of: _____

_____

_____

Ways I'd like to change my diet: _____

_____

_____

Specific foods I'd like to incorporate into my diet: _____

_____

_____

Factors that get in the way of me changing my diet: _____

_____

_____

Top two things that make it hardest for me to change my diet:

1. _____

_____

2. _____

_____

Strategies that I can use to overcome diet change barrier #1:

_____

_____

Strategies that I can use to overcome diet change barrier #2:

_____

_____

Small steps I can take to change my diet (even a little bit) this week: _____

_____

_____

Small steps I can take to change my diet (even a little bit) this month: _____

_____

_____

Dietary goals I have for myself over the next 3 months:

_____

_____

_____

Dietary goals I have for myself over the next 6 months:

_____

_____

_____

Things I've learned from this chapter that could help me change my diet: _____

_____

_____

How changing my diet is consistent with my current values:

_____

_____

_____

Sleep and the Advantages of a Well-Rested Brain

IN MY CLINICAL PRACTICE, SOMETIMES I SEE INDI-
viduals who feel that they're losing their ability to concentrate, reason, and remember in daily life, only to discover
that their lapses are likely related to sleep problems (and
not something like Alzheimer's disease). This issue comes
up across the entire life span. Some children and adolescents with suspected ADHD—including those who report
having problems with focus and organization—are actually struggling due to problems getting to sleep or staying asleep. While excessive social media use is sometimes
to blame, burdensome homework demands or an undiag-
nosed sleep disorder can be in the mix too. In adults and
older adults, sleep apnea may be leading to concentration
or memory difficulties that people mistakenly believe are
signs of impending dementia. Getting to the bottom of
what causes people's cognitive challenges is my job, and

sleep is one factor I routinely consider given its role in help-ing or harming brain health.

In this chapter, we'll drill down into the relationship between sleep and the brain. I consider this topic another part of the "P" (*prevention*) category of the C.A.P.E. model, in that maintaining healthy sleep levels can help prevent cog-nitive problems from occurring. Unfortunately, ongoing or poorly managed problems with sleep can negatively impact the brain, sometimes in significant ways. We also know that insomnia—a general term referring to problems maintain-ing sleep throughout the night—is one of various risk fac-tors for dementia and other cognitive problems. So, this is a topic we need to take very seriously in light of both positive and negative effects of sleep on the brain.

THE BACKGROUND SCIENCE

The sweet spot of sleep for most people is 7 to 8 hours per night. Being in this range most of the time is necessary for good health—general and brain-related. While many peo-ple sleep in the ideal 7- to 8-hour range, over 30% of people sleep more or less. As we'll discuss, both *short sleeping* (sleep-ing less than 6 hours) and *long sleeping* (sleeping more than 9 hours) can be problematic for the brain and body.

Curiously, a recent survey from the National Sleep Foun-dation found that 65% of American adults believe in the value of sleep to improve their own productivity, but only 10% said that they prioritize sleep in their daily lives. Huh?

Seems like a remarkable example of talking the talk but not walking the walk. We can all relate to occasional late nights for completing a work project or caring for a sick child, but to rank sleep lower than physical fitness, nutrition, work, and hobbies—also described in the study above—seems concerning. **Here, we'll consider the impact of sleep on brain and cognitive functioning, and I hope to convince you of the importance of putting sleep at or near the top of your own life-priorities list.**

How Sleep Helps the Brain Work Better

When we get down to the nitty-gritty details of sleep, what does it actually do for us? Scientists, philosophers, psychologists, physicians, and mystics have debated this topic for decades if not hundreds of years. The science, especially the most recent research, has helped clarify why sleep is so critically important for the body *and* the brain.

One of the most exciting developments in sleep neuroscience relates to a neuronal waste product called beta-amyloid. Beta-amyloid is a known contributor to Alzheimer's disease, and as it accumulates, it can lead to brain plaques and inflammation. So, the less of it we have circulating in the brain, the better. While beta-amyloid occurs naturally in the brain, problems start to crop up when there's more of it being created than disposed of.

We now know that sleep appears to flush beta-amyloid from the brain, helping rid the brain of this potentially toxic by-product. This occurs by way of the *glymphatic system*, the brain's internal cleanup crew, which is active almost exclusively when we're asleep. This doesn't necessarily mean that sleeping well will prevent dementia, but there seems to be something essential about catching our ZZZ's that reduces the negative impact of the brain's garbage.

Some recent research nails home this point: people who report poor sleep quality and sleepiness during the day have more Alzheimer's-like changes in the brain, including buildup of beta-amyloid in multiple areas linked to executive functioning and emotional regulation. We also see that over time, beta-amyloid accumulates faster in the brains of people who report lots of daytime sleepiness (an indication of poor nighttime sleep quality), potentially increasing their vulnerability to develop dementia.

Even more concerning is that people who sleep poorly have a higher risk of developing cognitive impairment and Alzheimer's disease—one large meta-analytic study found a 68% *higher risk* of mild to more severe cognitive problems. This level of risk relates to all types of sleep difficulties, although sleep apnea sets up a particular vulnerability for cognitive deficits. The researchers also found that sleep problems could potentially account for 15% of existing Alzheimer's disease cases. That's a huge number of people who may have been able to prevent this devastating condition with better management of sleep problems. Other evidence points to sleep disturbance interfering with frontal lobe functioning, which leads to difficulties with executive functions and mood regulation. The bottom line is that any and all sleep difficulties, especially if chronic and poorly managed, can deal a devastating blow to the brain.

The Long and the Short of It

Beyond something as concerning as dementia, sleeping too little—or too much—can cause milder cognitive challenges too. And this isn't necessarily in the context of a diagnosable sleep disorder per se. As one common example, perhaps you tend to curb sleep during the workweek, only to catch up on the weekend. Many people struggle to get all the sleep they need during the week due to ramped-up job demands, schedule changes, or child-care duties. The logic usually goes something like this: I'll lose a little sleep this week, but I'll sleep in on Saturday and Sunday and be fine by next week. Sound familiar?

Unfortunately, this logic doesn't work out so well according to sleep neuroscience. One well-conducted study looked at the effects of restricting sleep to 4 or 6 hours per night for a period of 2 weeks, or—the more extreme experimental condition—completely depriving people of sleep for 2 nights. The findings may serve as a wake-up call, pardon the pun, to those who try to catch up on sleep after a sleep-deprived workweek. The researchers found that sleeping 4 or 6 hours per night soon resulted in various cognitive deficits, including problems with sustained attention, working memory, and information processing speed. Another finding was also revealing: when people were restricted to 4 hours of nightly sleep over the course of 2 weeks, their thinking skills were just as impaired as those in people who were totally sleep deprived for 2 nights. In just a few days, sleeping less than 8 hours per night really hit the brain hard.

People who are *short sleepers* have another troubling tendency: they feel that their thinking skills are just fine, even though their cognitive performance indicates otherwise. Curiously, this tendency doesn't apply as much to people who go without a night of sleep—they realize they're wiped out, both physically and mentally. Your coworker who brags about not sleeping much while completing a project but still being on his game . . . well, he might be a tad mistaken on that assessment.

How about sleeping too much, also known as *long sleeping?* While there's nothing wrong with sleeping in from time to time, multiple studies have found that regularly sleeping more than 9 hours per night can have negative effects on problem-solving skills, language, and overall thinking ability. In industrialized nations, this is typically less common than short sleeping, but nevertheless carries a risk of cognitive difficulties if done often.

In terms of general health, short sleeping, particularly sleeping less than 6 hours per night, has been linked to a number of health problems, including an increased risk of diabetes, hypertension, heart disease, and obesity. Some of these conditions have been associated with long sleeping too. Given the problems with inadequate or excessive sleep for physical *and* brain health, finding ways to maintain the 7- to 8-hour sweet spot is all the more important. Next, we'll consider some strategies that can help.

Is Your Sleep "Hygienic"?

Sometimes sleep problems—including ones that negatively affect brain health—are related to how we wind down at the end of the day. The broad category of habits related to promoting sleep is what's called *sleep hygiene*. One important aspect of sleep hygiene is your bedtime routine. As you get ready to go to bed, are you staring at a screen, like your phone, TV, or a tablet? Or are you doing something relaxing, such as reading a book, taking a bath, or engaging in meditation? A consistent nighttime routine involving activities to quiet your body and mind can be helpful at kicking in your circadian rhythms and drifting away to a peaceful slumber.

A related point concerns the time at which we go to sleep and wake the next day. While not always possible, having consistent times when you get into bed and, hopefully 7 to 8 hours later, wake up to greet the day, can train your mind into recognizing when to wind down and when to start up again. Inconsistent sleep or wake times can throw your sleep cycle out of whack—including if you consistently sleep in much later on the weekend—and make it hard for your body to adjust to the time window when you sleep.

Do you notice a connection between what you've had to drink or eat and troubles getting to sleep? Caffeine is one of the main culprits in poor sleep quality. Having anything caffeinated in the afternoon—coffee, soda, even chocolate—can end up interfering with sleep. Eating spicy or fatty foods can also impact sleep for some people.

Another aspect of sleep hygiene involves the associations we have with our bed. Eating in bed, working in bed, and looking at screens in bed can train the brain into thinking that our bed is a multitasking zone rather than one reserved for relaxation (and intimacy). These associations can interfere with the sleep process, particularly in terms of how well we start the night's sleep.

Monitoring your own tendencies related to sleep hygiene (including with "The Brass Tacks" worksheet at the end of the chapter) might be illuminating. Habits that are out of our immediate awareness may have a clear relationship to the sleep challenges we experience. Fortunately, this means that as we become more aware of what we do in the minutes and hours before bedtime, we may discover a few things to change that allow us to get a bit more shut-eye.

The Joys (and Brain Health Benefits) of an Afternoon Snooze

How often do you take naps? While napping sometimes gets a bad rap, the science on napping and the brain indicates that it's a great strategy to promote brain health. In college, I had a boss who reliably took a 20-minute nap every day. He put a sticky note on his door with "ZZZ" written on it, alerting others to give him space for a few minutes. At the time, I thought this was an unusual habit for a working adult. But in retrospect, I get it—Dave was one of the most productive, hard-working people I've ever known. Outside of his nap time, he was engaged, energetic, and full of great (and actionable) ideas. We now know that the science clearly supports Dave's efforts and those of other regular nappers.

Simply put, napping has well-known positive effects on brain health. Some research has shown that naps can improve our executive functioning skills, especially working memory. Perhaps because of scaled-up working memory, we tend to learn information better after we take a nap. Naps also enhance our ability to consolidate, or lock in, new memories and may improve our ability to process emotionally charged information and manage stress. Lots of clear benefits here.

From a biological standpoint, neuroscience research has also shown that napping seems particularly helpful at clearing out *adenosine*, a so-called neuromodulator in the brain that builds up throughout the day and increases our sense of sleepiness. If you're a coffee drinker, you're already familiar with the effects of adenosine; caffeine reduces the impact of adenosine on the brain, helping improve our alertness. There's also evidence that napping reduces inflammation caused by the body's immune system; we've discussed inflammation throughout the book as a response from the body that is linked to brain problems.

How long you nap also matters. Studies indicate that naps

of less than 30 minutes—the classic power nap—seem to be associated with the best cognitive and health outcomes. The sweet spot might even be 10 to 20 minutes, particularly in terms of improved alertness and processing speed after the nap. Note that this brain boost occurs once the mild sluggishness after a nap, referred to as sleep inertia, wears off. It also seems that napping in the afternoon, particularly in the early afternoon, promotes our cognitive skills better than in the morning.

Now, all naps are not created equal. Napping can be helpful for brain and overall health when you get the ideal 7 to 8 hours of sleep at night. However, the need to take naps more frequently can be a clear indicator of nighttime sleep problems. Further, people who consistently nap longer than 30 minutes (especially 60+ minutes) are less likely to have lasting benefits and are more prone to depression, cardiovascular disease, or other health problems. Longer naps may also disrupt the sleep cycle. Your body can lose some of the urgency to sleep around bedtime after a long nap, disrupting the ability to initiate and maintain sleep through the night. So, treading lightly with naps seems to be a good way to go for general and brain-related health.

Purpose and Gratitude

Sometimes in the research world, people uncover relationships between variables that are quite unexpected or, at the very least, not intuitive at first pass. **This subsection** describes the science related to two topics you may not have anticipated reading about in a chapter on sleep: purpose in life and gratitude.

People with a distinct purpose in life—a sense of meaning and conviction that helps guide one's actions—tend to live longer and have a lower risk of problems like stroke, mild cognitive impairment, and Alzheimer's disease. But did you know that a sense of life purpose is also related to your sleep quality? Believe it or not, multiple studies have clarified this connection. One 4-year study looked at sleep problems and purpose in life in a group of over 4,000 people. Not an easy study to conduct given the number of participants and the length of time they were followed. People answered questionnaires that asked about general health problems, emotional concerns, sleep difficulties, and purpose in life (for the latter measure, there were questions like, "I have a sense of direction and purpose in my life").

The researchers found that people who had a sense of purpose in life reported considerably fewer sleep problems. Those with the strongest sense of purpose had the best sleep quality; each uptick on the life-purpose measure was linked to a 16% lower chance of sleep challenges. Since the study was designed to account for confounding issues that might have influenced study results (for example, depression, anxiety, and medical problems), it seems likely that one's sense of purpose truly is linked to how well or poorly one sleeps.

Other work has found that leading a purposeful life reduces the risk of sleep-related disorders like sleep apnea or restless legs syndrome. One possibility is that when you feel your life has a meaningful direction, you're motivated to make better lifestyle choices—eating well, exercising, staying socially engaged—and this includes efforts to prioritize sleep to improve overall health.

Another thing you wouldn't necessarily associate with your sleep satisfaction: how often you express gratitude in daily life. Gratitude has gotten lots of attention over the past few years in the scientific community for its powerful effects on resilience and general wellness. Some studies have also demonstrated its influence on how we sleep. For example, when people engage in gratitude exercises—like regularly recording what they're grateful for in a diary—they report improved sleep quality. This has been shown to occur over short periods of time, suggesting that even small tweaks to your daily routine could have important effects on your sleep (and quality of life).

While it's unclear why showing gratitude improves sleep quality, there's some evidence that people have fewer troubling thoughts at night when they engage in grateful gestures. Perhaps reflecting on what's good in our lives reduces the mental chatter that creeps in when we feel burdened by stress and daily challenges.

The Special Case of Sleep Apnea

Sleep-related breathing problems, primarily obstructive sleep apnea (OSA), are fairly common. OSA becomes more common in middle age and often occurs in older adults: up to 50% of men and 25% of women. This condition can result in dozens if not hundreds of "hypoxic" episodes—brief periods where the brain is deprived of oxygen—throughout the night. **A number of my patients have been alarmed to learn that sleep apnea can affect brain structure and cognitive function fairly significantly, especially if it goes untreated.**

Why this occurs is somewhat unclear, although scientists have proposed and investigated several possibilities. One is that lingering effects of sleepiness during the day due to poor sleep the night before results in slower processing speed, weaker attention, and diminished memory. There is some evidence supporting this hypothesis, although even when people report less sleepiness due to effective treatment of OSA, they can still exhibit memory and other cognitive problems.

Another hypothesis is that the various hypoxic episodes caused by OSA result in lasting damage to the brain. Some structures in the brain, including the memory-critical hippocampus, are particularly vulnerable to oxygen deprivation. OSA has been found to shrink the hippocampus and have negative effects on other structures such as the amygdala, thalamus, and frontal lobes.

Not all people with sleep apnea have cognitive lapses. But for those who do, concentration and memory are commonly affected. Information processing speed and visual–spatial abilities can take a hit. We see problems with multiple executive functioning skills like problem solving, working memory, and flexible thinking. Sleep researchers have also discovered that people with sleep-disordered breathing experience cognitive changes (including dementia) earlier than others.

Fortunately, using a continuous positive airway pressure (CPAP) device can mitigate these changes. This device provides continuous air pressure while sleeping, minimizing if not eliminating the many apneic episodes throughout the night. People consistently using CPAP show improved thinking skills in multiple areas including memory, attention, and executive functioning. However, depending on how severe the sleep apnea is and how long it's been untreated, some cognitive deficits may persist.

Getting a sleep evaluation for persistent sleep problems is quite important, as related treatment can protect your brain from further changes and potentially reverse those that have already occurred.

Does the Early Bird Really Get the Worm?

You may have heard about a hot topic in the sleep world: delaying school start times for adolescents. Teenagers tend to go to sleep later than kids in elementary and middle school, but it's not just because of ubiquitous screens and social media: **the teen brain experiences some notable shifts that affect sleep.** The circadian rhythms change in such a way that teens have less of an urge to sleep until later in the evening. Melatonin, which also contributes to sleepiness, takes longer to get secreted in the teen brain and body, further delaying sleep onset.

Because of these biological changes, teenagers who start school particularly early tend to sleep much less than they should, the ideal amount for teens being 8.5 to 9.5 hours per night. The result: School districts with earlier starts (generally defined as 8 AM or earlier) have students who struggle with a wide variety of academic, cognitive, and emotional problems. These include lower grades, weaker concentration and executive functioning, disciplinary issues, and depression. Even driving is affected. Teen drivers in school districts with earlier start times are at a much higher risk of being in a vehicular accident. This could be due to the negative effects of sleep deprivation on information processing speed; sleepy teens are slower to react on the road.

In contrast, research has also shown that the later schools begin classes, the more sleep students get, and the more likely students will respond favorably in a variety of ways. Perhaps it goes without saying that they tend to be more alert and attentive in class when they're well rested. They attend school more consistently, get better grades, have higher scores on standardized tests like the SAT, and drive more safely. There's also evidence that kids in delayed-start districts have better interactions within their family and have fewer emotional and behavioral problems.

Large associations, including the American Psychological Association, American Academy of Pediatrics, and American Medical Association, have recommended that schools start at 8:30 AM or later given the many benefits to additional sleep. While there can be administrative and logistical challenges when implementing delayed-start times, Dr. William Kobler of the American Medical Association clarified the bottom line related to this issue: "The health benefits for adolescents far outweigh any potential negative consequences." Many school districts across the country have heeded this advice. Perhaps this is a topic to raise at your own school board meeting given the important implications for adolescents' brain health and general wellness.

THE BOTTOM LINE

I hope you've learned some new things related to sleep and brain health; here are a few key points to keep in mind:

- The ideal window for sleep duration for most people is 7 to 8 hours per night.
- Sleeping less than 6 hours per night—short sleeping— is associated with multiple cognitive problems, including reduced attention, working memory, and processing speed.
- Sleeping more than 9 hours per night—long sleeping— can also cause cognitive difficulties.
- Short sleeping during the workweek and long sleeping to "catch up" on the weekend is risky from a cognitive standpoint.
- Sleep hygiene strategies, such as avoiding caffeine in

the afternoon, not watching TV or other screens in bed, doing something relaxing before bed, and having consistent sleep and wake-up times, can help promote healthy and satisfying sleep.

- Expressing gratitude and having a clear sense of purpose in life can positively affect your sleep quality.
- Naps less than 30 minutes, particularly in the afternoon, can enhance cognitive abilities such as working memory, learning, and memory consolidation.
- Sleep apnea, especially when left untreated, can negatively impact multiple cognitive skills including attention, processing speed, memory, and executive functioning.
- Use of a CPAP device to treat sleep apnea can lead to cognitive improvement.
- High school students who start classes at 8:30 AM or later do better in their classes, are more emotionally healthy, and get in fewer car accidents.

THE BRASS TACKS:
PERSONAL STRATEGIC PLANNING
TO IMPROVE MY SLEEP

I would describe my sleep now as (check one):

____ Good; essentially no problems

____ Occasional problems

____ A fair amount of problems

____ Lots of problems

I typically feel rested with the amount of sleep I get (circle one):   Y   N

Amount of sleep I usually get each night: _____

Each week, I have trouble with my sleep (check one):

_____ Less than once per week

_____ About once per week

_____ 2 to 3 days per week

_____ 4 or more days per week

Sleep hygiene factors that could interfere with my sleep (watching a screen before bed; consuming something caffeinated, fatty, or spicy late in the day; inconsistent bedtime or wake up time; and so on): _____

_____

_____

Top two things I could try to improve my sleep habits/ hygiene and quality:

1. _____

_____

2. _____

_____

Strategies that I can use to implement #1: _____

_____

_____

Strategies that I can use to implement #2: _____

_____

_____

Small steps I can take to sleep better (even a little bit) this week: _____

_____

_____

Small steps I can take to sleep better (even a little bit) this month: _____

_____

_____

Sleep goals I have for myself over the next 3 months:

_____

_____

_____

Sleep goals I have for myself over the next 6 months:

_____

_____

_____

Things I've learned from this chapter that could help me improve my sleep: _____

_____

_____

How improving my sleep is consistent with my current values:

_____

_____

_____

Mellowing the Stressed-Out Brain

STRESS IS PART OF LIFE. WE ALL HAVE DEADLINES, projects, social interactions, or upcoming events that stress us out. Benjamin Franklin was onto something when he proclaimed that the only certainties in life were death and taxes; I would add that the experience of being frazzled or overwhelmed by something is a universal experience too.

When I see people for cognitive evaluations, sometimes I find that the main cause of memory problems they report is not a brain-related disorder. **Stress has such a powerful influence on our mood and thinking skills that it alone can explain why some folks feel like they can't seem to focus or remember things well.**

As one example, Alex was a father of two whose work in sales intensified after a recent promotion to a managerial role. Despite being thrilled to move up the ranks in his company, he felt like he couldn't concentrate on tasks or recall what he recently learned. When he saw his primary-care doctor, his score on a brief cognitive screening measure was normal, despite having cognitive complaints in daily life. In my work with him, he reported moderate symptoms of anxiety (which he attributed to his stress), but performed fine on tests of memory, concentration, and problem solving. He was receptive to developing better stress-management strategies, and was reassured to learn that he did not have a brain-related disorder. We also discussed the impact that stress can have on our efficiency and productivity for reasons I'll review below.

As another aspect of the "P" for *prevention* in the C.A.P.E. model, effectively managing stress is a powerful way to prevent cognitive problems. Acute stress can temporarily hijack our brain; chronic stress can lead to problems with multiple thinking skills and literally shrink brain structures. **Fortunately, having a good stress-management "toolbox" on hand can promote brain health and quality of life.** Let's start with what the science says about stress and the brain.

THE BACKGROUND SCIENCE

Day-to-day stress is something we all experience. Feeling overwhelmed at work or home, struggling to pay the bills, having challenging interactions with coworkers or family members: these all count. Stress is hard to define specifically, but we know it when we see (or feel) it. It's also safe to say that what's stressful for one person is stimulating for another. Public speaking is a classic example: some people love getting up in front of others and teaching what they know. Others would rather have a root canal.

Our sense of stress also changes over time. What was stressful at one point earlier in life may no longer be a concern now. Some people hate parallel parking when they learn to drive but later enjoy the puzzle of fitting their car just right into the only available spot. Trying many things the first time can be frustrating, embarrassing, even agonizing; after we practice a bit, we shed the stress and replace it with more positive feelings.

The science of stress has important implications for the practicalities of managing challenges in daily life. Stress research may also seem counterintuitive at first pass. Take the classic Yerkes–Dodson law of stress (Figure 10.1).

The Yerkes–Dodson law is the most enduring description of the stress response—it's been around for decades—

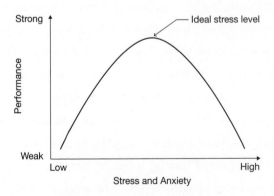

FIGURE 10.1 Yerkes–Dodson Law of Stress

Image adapted from Fig. 2, p. 250, in D.O. Hebb (1955), Drives and the C.N.S., Psychological Review, 62(4), 243–254. Content in public domain.

and one that remains relevant for our purposes here. **The main takeaway from this concept is that some stress is actually a *good* thing. The problem is when stress ramps up and overwhelms us, or when we feel an absence of stress and get bored.** Moderate levels of stress activate and mobilize us to take action. Think about how an upcoming deadline kicks our planning and organization into gear, or how a presentation in front of colleagues inspires more intense efforts to plan out the key points. We refer to the varied levels of stress as an *inverted U-shaped curve*: a little or a lot is bad, a moderate amount right in the middle is ideal.

When stress becomes particularly intense, it's no longer serving a useful purpose. This is when we become scattered, anxious, and classically stressed out. As we discussed earlier in the book, there's a whimsical but descriptive term coined by psychologist Daniel Goleman that applies to this negative state: the *amygdala hijack*. Excessive stress, combined with difficulties applying strategies to reduce it, causes some brain regions to use more physiological resources than usual. The amygdala—the brain's fire alarm that goes off when there is a perceived threat of some sort—will actually override the rational problem-solving frontal lobes when stress moves into the danger zone. In fact, some research has shown that the connection between the amygdala and the frontal lobes is essentially severed during stressful states, making it hard to think and reason effectively. The goal, of course, is to cool down the amygdala so that the frontal cortex can reengage. While easier said than done, later we'll consider some simple yet powerful strategies along these lines that can really cut the stress response.

Another key point to consider is that the stress we feel is based on how we perceive and *appraise* the stressor in question. One of the common maxims of stress: a given situation or activity is ultimately less important than how we personally interpret its meaningfulness. This is actually the foundation of a type of psychotherapy called cognitive–behavioral therapy, the idea being that our emotions (including those generated by stress) are directly related to our thoughts and beliefs. Optimistic thoughts lead to positive emotions; negative thoughts can hijack our brains and cause anxiety, stress, and depression.

The stress-induced amygdala hijack has its roots in a larger system in the brain and body called the hypothalamic–pituitary–adrenal (HPA) axis. This system helps us quickly react to and mobilize for an environmental threat by releasing two key stress hormones: adrenaline and cortisol. Once these hormones are circulating, the body responds through the classic *fight-or-flight response*. Fifty thousand years ago, this response might have led to throwing a spear at the saber-toothed tiger behind the bush . . . or running like heck to safety.

Fast forward to the present day, and the same physiological reaction can be problematic for the brain and body, particularly when we experience stress day in and day out. Rather than a ferocious predator, the "threat" in our environment could be a hostile e-mail, a damning glance in the hall from a coworker, or a heated discussion with a partner. To the brain, though, these experiences are equivalent, activating the stress response and potentially leading to prolonged negative feelings.

Stressed Out and Cognitively Challenged

Stress and cognitive abilities don't mix well. The cortisol released during the stress response gets us ready for action, but it can also do nasty things to the brain if the stress continues. In fact, too much cortisol can negatively affect multiple cognitive skills such as processing speed, memory, and executive functioning. Over the long haul, cortisol is neurotoxic—it literally kills neurons—and can even shrink multiple brain regions. The hippocampus is one of the areas most affected by stress, which can translate into memory lapses during stressful periods. The hippocampus is particularly vulnerable because it has lots of glucocorticoid receptors, which are parts of neurons that cortisol gloms onto. The frontal lobes are full of the same types of receptors, which is one reason why stress can impair our executive skills too.

One of the key executive functions we rely on in daily life—mental flexibility, or the ability to consider or create new solutions on the fly—is particularly impacted by stress. Consider how important this ability is. When was the last time you needed to change your schedule because of something unexpected? Or while driving, you came to a major construction detour, and you needed to figure out a new route? Or when you realized that someone's perspective, though different than yours, had merit and needed further consideration? When under stress, we become more fixed, even rigid in how we see things. This can interfere with decisions we need to make or the interactions we have with others.

Some research has looked at how stress in the moment affects our thinking skills. One study had people engage in two activities that many people consider stressful. First, they had to give a speech describing their interest in joining a law office or being admitted to business school. Then they had to do mental arithmetic problems for 5 minutes. And how's this for a good time: both of these tasks were done in front of a panel of scientists in lab coats who were taking notes and giving no overt signs of approval. The study participants were also being video and audio recorded and were told that their performance was going to be analyzed later by experts. Not exactly a warm and fuzzy environment.

During the experiment, people would be interrupted and asked to complete tests of problem solving and creativity, such as unscrambling mixed-up words as quickly as possible (easier said than done). This would happen to folks in the "stress" condition of the experiment and to those in the "control" condition, who had been doing something fairly benign like reading a passage or counting out loud in an empty room. The research revealed that when people felt stressed out, they had significantly more trouble thinking flexibly: it was much harder for them to unscramble words, and they also took more time to solve problems they were presented with. Curiously, other abilities, including visual memory and fine motor coordination, weren't affected by stress. It seems that feeling stressed has a particularly negative effect on some of our essential executive functioning skills.

Beth was a patient of mine who was concerned about her problems remembering information in the moment, such as learning names of new people she met or recalling why she walked into a certain room in her house. She was also under a great deal of stress due to being laid off from her job (yet another victim of corporate downsizing) and related financial struggles. Fortunately, her neuropsychological evaluation results indicated that her cognitive abilities were largely intact, with only a few subtle weaknesses.

I told her that her psychosocial stress was likely affecting her working memory—how well she could hold onto and manipulate information in her mind for short periods of time—and that she would probably experience improvement once things in her life stabilized (like securing a new job). As we considered in Chapter 3, what we describe as "memory problems" can actually mean lots of things. In Beth's case, she was having mild difficulties with working memory but not with other memory subtypes like episodic or semantic memory.

As Beth can attest, working memory is another executive function heavily impacted by stress. Some research has found that stress interferes with remembering information for brief periods, but it doesn't necessarily affect other aspects of memory. Stress may distract us in the moment, but it doesn't always impair our memory for new material.

A broader perspective is that stressful experiences, particularly ones where we don't feel like we're in control of the situation, affect the executive functions and their neurological home, the brain's frontal cortex. As we've discussed, we see this in terms of reduced mental flexibility and working memory; problems can also take the form of reacting more impulsively when we're under stress (like abusing substances or overeating).

Earlier we considered the inverted U-shaped curve from the Yerkes–Dodson law that depicted the effects of stress on performance, where too much *or* too little stress is a bad thing. The best place is right in between—just enough stress to keep us motivated and engaged. The plot thickens when we consider why this inverted U-shaped curve describes stress levels so well. It seems that levels of two neurotransmitters—dopamine and norepinephrine—help determine the extent to which stress affects our cognitive abilities. An overabundance of these brain chemicals can lead us to react negatively to something and impair our frontal lobe functioning, particularly our working memory. Not enough can be associated with us feeling sluggish and bored. Notably, the main stress hormone—cortisol—also tends to follow the same inverted U-shaped curve.

One study considered a situation that many of us would describe as pretty stressful: preparing for a major exam.

Stressed-out medical students—studying for a medical licensing exam—were asked to shift their attention from one thing to another while their brain activity was being monitored with functional magnetic resonance imaging (fMRI) brain scans. When the students were compared to other people not in the process of studying (and who were understandably less stressed), they were found to have much more trouble focusing. Even more concerning, multiple brain areas were less connected than usual: the frontal lobes of the anxious students were communicating poorly with the parietal lobes and a few other regions. The researchers argued that the students' stress had caused their frontal lobes to short-circuit and not link up as well with other parts of the brain.

But get this: About a month after the board exam, when the students were more relaxed—lo and behold—their brain functioning normalized. The students' frontal lobes recovered their connections with other regions and essentially returned to their non-stressed state. This study clarified what most people can relate to: under stress, we can feel like we're losing our marbles! The science clearly indicates that the stress response can really mess with our brains when it's present, particularly affecting the frontal lobes and executive functions. After the stress has subsided, we regain our composure, and, more generally, we feel like ourselves again.

Note that brain rewiring due to stress is a good example of *plasticity*. The brain changes with experience in both positive and negative ways, and these changes are not necessarily permanent (including the negative ones, fortunately). Unlike what early neuroscientists said years ago, the brain is not set in stone after early development; rather, it's always in motion throughout life, being swayed to and fro by experiences of all sorts.

The Enduring Effects of Stress

We know from our discussion so far that brief periods of stress can do troubling things to some of our thinking skills, particularly the executive functions. But what about stress that piles up over time? **Not surprisingly, chronic stress can have additional negative effects on how the brain looks and operates.** A few particularly revealing studies have clarified the brain-related burdens of ongoing stress.

Some research has looked at the frequency of stressful life events across a few months—things like financial problems, losing a job, or the end of an important relationship—and the brain. In one study, the more stress people experienced over a 3-month period, *the smaller multiple brain regions became.* The areas with less brain mass due to stress included the memory-powerhouse hippocampus and the concentration-promoting cingulate cortex. So, it certainly makes sense that people under chronic stress report problems learning and remembering new things; the parts of the brain associated with these abilities literally shrink when under stress, probably due to the toxic effects of cortisol.

In a related vein, a longitudinal study considered the

effects of stress on the brain over a 20-year period. The researchers asked a group of women to rate their perceived stress every year or two, and then after two decades they underwent brain MRI scans. At that point, the researchers attempted to understand the role of chronic stress on the brain by correlating the women's stress ratings with the size of different brain regions. The study revealed that more reported stress was associated with reduced brain volume in parts of the hippocampus and a frontal lobe region (the orbitofrontal cortex), suggesting a very real brain-based effect of ongoing stress.

Other research has concluded essentially the same thing, particularly regarding the detrimental effects of chronic stress on multiple areas within the prefrontal cortex. And in adults in their sixties, those reporting high levels of stress over the course of a decade are *about 40% more likely to be diagnosed with mild cognitive impairment* than people experiencing less stress. It perhaps goes without saying that stress clearly wreaks havoc on the body and the brain if not managed appropriately in the moment and over the years.

Science has also clarified that even a single stressful or traumatic event can have an ongoing impact on the brain. For example, one study looked at individuals who were within 1.5 miles of the 9/11 World Trade Center terrorist attack. More than 3 years later, people who were close to the site of the attack had less brain volume in several areas— the hippocampus, the amygdala, and parts of the prefrontal cortex—compared to people who lived hundreds of miles away. Note that the people close to the attack did not have a psychological condition such as post-traumatic stress disorder (PTSD), so a more severe outcome like that couldn't explain the findings. Just being exposed to such a distressing experience altered the brain.

It's also important to acknowledge that reduced brain volume as seen in acute and chronic stress doesn't necessarily translate into weaker cognitive abilities. This may occur in some people, but others continue to function just fine cognitively. All else being equal, though, more brain mass is ideal. Less gray matter can set up a vulnerability to develop not only cognitive difficulties, but psychological ones too. For example, we know that conditions such as mood and anxiety disorders are associated with less volume in the same brain regions we've discussed that are affected by stress. **In the interest of potentially reversing or altogether preventing these problems, next we'll review the science related to reducing stress and rejuvenating the brain.**

Stress-Busting Strategies

While hiking in a magnificent redwood forest with my wife, I was awestruck by both the splendor of these natural giants and the trees that seemed to define resilience in the face of remarkable adversity. The bases of many trees were almost completely hollowed out due to wildfires, lightning strikes, fungus, and efforts from opportunistic animals to take shelter. What was particularly impressive was the ability of the redwoods not only to survive these destructive blows, but also to rebound and continue to grow, sometimes hundreds of feet in the air. A flourishing redwood is a useful metaphor for stress management that we all aspire to: successfully coping with challenges in daily life so that we learn and grow in the face of stress.

You've probably heard of mindfulness, or more specifically, mindfulness meditation. This stress-management and relaxation strategy comes in different forms but essentially revolves around the notion of remaining present, reflective, and non-judgmental in any given moment. Mindfulness has been described extensively in the popular media. It's also a common strategy used in business settings, large and small, to help people manage their stress and stay focused at work and in general. Trends in mental health come and go (sometimes for good reason), but mindfulness has stood the test of time. This is partly because it's already been around for a while—something on the order of a few thousand years.

There are various types of mindfulness exercises one can engage in. A common one is simply attending to your breath. Try this for a moment: get into a comfortable seated position, and then inhale slowly to a count of three, paying attention to the fresh air filling your lungs. Hold your breath for a second, then exhale to a count of three, attending to the air and stress that are leaving your body. Try that cycle a few times (perhaps 8 to 10 repetitions), all the while imaging the benefits of the air you're breathing and the tension you're releasing with each exhalation. At the same time, be aware of, but don't judge the thoughts coming into your mind. These will come and go; just mentally observe them without devoting too much time to them.

You can also take on a mundane task in a mindful way. For example, most people don't like doing the dishes or the laundry, although both offer an opportunity to focus in the moment on the details of an activity that might otherwise go unnoticed. When doing the dishes, attend to the sound of the water on the plate you're washing; deliberately scrub away the leftover salad dressing or lasagna cheese with mindful effort, focusing on each swipe with the scrubber brush. When pulling clothes from the dryer, rather than rushing through the perceived time sink of this activity, consider folding each item with intention, sleeve by sleeve, pant leg by pant leg. This is the essence of mindfulness: everything we do offers an opportunity to remain in the moment.

Even attending to a specific sense—part of what's called *effortless awareness*—can improve our ability to be mindful of our experience. This involves simply being aware of the sense that we're using most in any given moment, such as what we're hearing or seeing. Our prominent sense can shift frequently, and by observing our senses in this way, we can often tune out stress and tune in to ourselves.

These sorts of exercises can help reduce stress in the moment. Over time, they can also enhance cognitive health and help the brain regain some of its mass that stress pre-

viously shrunk. Something else to keep in mind: meditation, broadly speaking, helps promote richer connections
throughout and across each of the brain's hemispheres,
potentially leading to better information processing and
improvement in other cognitive skills. And we know that
certain types of mindfulness—such as simply labeling our
emotional states—can kick the frontal lobes into gear and
reestablish their control over the mercurial amygdala.

There's a specific training program related to mindfulness
—Mindfulness-Based Stress Reduction, or MBSR—that
may be available in your area. I mention this because it's a
really good way to learn more about mindfulness if you're
interested. It has also specifically been found to promote
brain health.

Remember how we discussed the parts of the brain that
are negatively affected by stress? MBSR essentially reverses
this process: it has been found to positively influence the
brain by increasing the size of multiple regions after just
a few months of training. One study had people engage in
MBSR for 8 weeks. At the end of the study, the research
participants improved their ability to focus in the moment,
meditate more effectively, and do mindful yoga. They also
had made their brains more robust: as a function of learning
MBSR and becoming more mindful, their left hippocampus
and posterior cingulate cortex got significantly larger. The
posterior cingulate cortex is associated with introspection
and self-reflection, so this brain change mirrored the skills
taught in MBSR. And we've discussed the importance of

the hippocampus for memory: the left side of this important structure is particularly crucial for verbal memory. It's also linked to our ability to regulate our emotions, which similarly tends to improve when we meditate.

Earlier we reviewed effortless awareness—a mindfulness meditation technique related to homing in on a specific sense, like what we're looking at or listening to. Some research has examined this strategy and its effects on the brain. One study compared experienced effortless-awareness meditators to novice meditators who were just getting started. It turns out that the expert meditators showed more *integration* throughout the brain; that is, multiple brain regions were better connected to each other. This might explain a finding from other studies showing that meditators tend to be effective at maintaining their focus for extended periods. Sustained attention requires coordination of multiple brain regions, so there seems to be something in the physiological "sauce" of meditation that helps promote this fundamental cognitive skill.

Yoga is another stress-management and general-wellness activity that has become increasingly popular in recent years. It's also sometimes included in studies examining mindfulness as one component of a relaxation "intervention." As we discussed earlier, yoga has some powerful effects on the brain. One recent study examined people who had consistently practiced yoga for 3 or more years. These practitioners showed significant brain-related differences compared to people who didn't do yoga: their verbal-memory-critical left hippocampus was larger, and their frontal lobes were more efficient when completing a working memory test. In a related vein, yoga practice is linked to benefits for cognitive skills like attention, processing speed, episodic memory, and executive functioning.

Remember in Chapter 3 when we did the self-affirmation exercise, where you indicated values that are particularly meaningful to you? It turns out that affirming what's important to you increases your ability to incorporate new habits into your life and put things in broader perspective. This introspective exercise can also help reduce stress.

A powerful study a few years ago asked a group of college students to determine their top two personal values and priorities (such as independence, creativity, or relationships with others) and write essays on why these were important to them. People in the control group wrote about their least important values and why these values might be important to others besides themselves. In other words, they engaged in some reflective analysis but not self-affirmation per se. Both groups were under quite a bit of stress, as they had particularly difficult midterm exams coming up. The researchers also considered whether people felt that their self-worth was at risk and whether they thought others would judge them negatively if they got a bad test score. Their stress was measured by self-report and also by a few common biological by-products of stress (urinary epinephrine and norepinephrine).

The findings revealed that the self-affirmation exercise before midterms really worked. People who wrote about their strongest values showed no increase in stress by-products during the study—from 2 weeks before the midterm exam to the day of the test—while the control group clearly did. The researchers also found that those who felt most personally threatened by the possibility of a bad test grade were most protected from stress by the self-affirmation exercise. Reflecting on our own values, even with a brief exercise like the one in this study, pays many psychological dividends. This seems to be the case in general and particularly when we feel vulnerable due to a stressful situation.

Positive psychology is the branch of psychology that studies uplifting human qualities such as optimism, happiness, and resilience. Related research on gratitude dovetails with our discussion of stress-management strategies. In one study, people were asked to write in a diary about things they were grateful for three times per week for 2 weeks. The researchers then rated lifestyle factors like the participants' sense of well-being and their sleep quality. Beyond improvement in sleep, people engaging in the gratitude exercise reported feeling more optimistic and having a better sense of well-being. Their blood pressure went down too. So, this brief gratitude intervention had far-reaching effects that were felt both psychologically and biologically. More generally, studies like this suggest that some types of self-reflection—like writing down what we're grateful for at least a few times per week—can improve our quality of life and stress management in a variety of ways. It also doesn't take long to experience the benefits of small but positive lifestyle changes.

It goes without saying that topics we've covered at other points in the book certainly help with stress management and, in turn, brain functioning. Staying socially and mentally engaged, eating well, and getting 7 to 8 hours of sleep per night all matter. Our discussion of exercise and the brain mostly focused on promoting brain and cognitive health; exercise is also one of the best stress-management strategies out there. People who are more physically active (either through aerobic activity or weight training) tend to report better emotional functioning, including fewer problems with stress and depression. Moving forward, perhaps you can add exercise and other ideas we've discussed to your stress-management "toolbox" in the interest of better physical, emotional, and brain-related health.

THE BOTTOM LINE

Here are a few particularly important takeaways related to stress and brain health:

- Experiences one person considers stressful are less stressful or even joyful to others.
- What's stressful at one point in time may be experienced very differently over time or after practice.

- Stress interferes with the workings of the hippocampus, which can lead to problems learning new information or recalling something you already know.
- Stress also affects the frontal lobes, which can translate into difficulties with working memory and flexible thinking.
- Stress can impact our cognitive skills over brief and extended periods of time.
- Mindfulness can be practiced at any moment: while breathing, doing the dishes, or taking care of the laundry.
- Consistently engaging in mindfulness exercises can strengthen the brain, particularly the hippocampus and frontal lobes.
- Yoga practice can expand some brain regions and improve cognitive abilities like attention and processing speed.
- Regularly affirming your most important personal values can significantly reduce your stress levels.
- In addition to its brain-boosting properties, exercise is an excellent stress-management strategy that improves emotional health.

THE BRASS TACKS:
PERSONAL STRATEGIC PLANNING TO
ACHIEVE MY STRESS-MANAGEMENT GOALS

Top three challenges or stressors in my life that are causing me stress:

1. _____

_____

2. _____

_____

3. _____

_____

Stressor #1 current severity rating (0 to 10 scale, from not severe to very severe; circle one):

0   1   2   3   4   5   6   7   8   9   10

Stressor #2 current severity rating (0 to 10 scale, from not severe to very severe; circle one):

0   1   2   3   4   5   6   7   8   9   10

Stressor #3 current severity rating (0 to 10 scale, from not severe to very severe; circle one):

0   1   2   3   4   5   6   7   8   9   10

Barriers that prevent me from reducing the impact of the stressors I listed above:

_____

_____

_____

Ways I can move beyond or manage these barriers: _____

_____

_____

Stress-reduction techniques and strategies that I'd like to try (or restart if I've tried something in the past): _____

_____

_____

Small steps I can take to reduce my stress (even a little bit) this week: _____

_____

_____

Small steps I can take to reduce my stress (even a little bit) this month: _____

_____

_____

Stress-management goals I have for myself over the next 3 months: _____

_____

_____

Stress-management goals I have for myself over the next 6 months: _____

_____

_____

Things I've learned from this chapter that could help me improve my stress management: _____

_____

_____

How managing stress better is consistent with my current values: _____

_____

_____

_____

11

Do Medical Problems and Smoking Affect How My Brain Works?

PAUL WAS DIAGNOSED WITH DIABETES IN HIS FIF-
ties and struggled to keep his blood sugar on track. While he tested his glucose levels fairly regularly, sometimes a few days passed without a check, and occasionally those checks revealed a distressingly out-of-kilter reading. He also used his medication inconsistently, a concern that his doctor and wife both raised with him. He was somewhat overweight but didn't otherwise have any diagnosed medical or psychological problems.

When he came in for a neuropsychological evaluation, he told me that his concentration and memory skills seemed to be slipping. The testing we did found some mild problems with his processing speed and his ability to learn new information. He actually retained new material pretty well once he had learned it, but he struggled to encode it in the first place. When we discussed the test findings, he was surprised to learn—as my diabetic patients often are—that diabetes can contribute to cognitive lapses.

In this chapter, we'll cover another aspect of the "P," or *prevention*, part of the C.A.P.E. model as it relates to medical problems and smoking. Specific medical problems covered here include diabetes, high blood pressure, and obesity, all of which are known to diminish brain health if not managed appropriately. Unfortunately, some people do all the right things to manage these conditions but still struggle to keep them under control. Other times, factors such as inconsistent medication compliance, lack of physical activity, and poor dietary choices can make medical problems much worse *and* negatively affect the brain. We also know that smoking can really do a number on the brain, particularly if someone has an underlying medical issue.

We'll talk about each of these areas in the context of brain health, with two goals: (1) clarify the impact of these so-called *cardiovascular risk factors* on our thinking skills, and (2) consider strategies to reduce their impact on the brain. Managing these issues even somewhat better can lead to improved general health and a better working brain.

THE BACKGROUND SCIENCE
Diabetes and the Brain

Cognitive challenges that occur in Paul's type of diabetes—*type 2 diabetes*, or what is often described as *adult-onset diabetes*—have been researched quite a bit. It turns out that diabetes can lead to problems with a few key thinking skills. One is cognitive processing speed, or how quickly you can manage and digest new information. Executive functioning and learning new material can also be reduced in diabetics. Over the course of time, people with diabetes tend to show increased difficulties with conversational word-finding too.

If you have diabetes or have been tested for it, you're probably familiar with your HbA1c levels. HbA1c, more commonly referred to as A1c, reflects your blood sugar levels over the past few months. Daily blood sugar readings, as measured by a finger-prick test, are much more variable than A1c levels, so doctors often look at A1c as a stable index of how well your diabetes is being controlled. Higher A1c levels put people at risk of additional medical issues, such as stroke, kidney problems, or damage to the eyes. They can also be linked to diminished brain health.

One recent study followed thousands of diabetics over the course of about 10 years, paying particular attention to their A1c levels and cognitive abilities. The researchers found that over time, people with higher A1c levels showed more significant cognitive decline in two areas: verbal memory and executive functioning. The executive skill that was reduced is what's called verbal fluency, measured by determining how many animals people could name in a minute. Note that performance on this test often relates to day-to-day struggles finding the right word to use in conversation. Also keep in mind that the study's findings were not related to other medical or emotional problems, indicating that fluctuating blood sugar in and of itself was linked to decreased thinking skills.

Of course, not everyone with diabetes has these sorts of difficulties, but diabetics are at heightened risk of experiencing them. It's also important to point out that cognitive problems that occur in diabetes are often in the mild—rather than moderate or severe—range. In other words, there may be changes that are noticeable and troubling, but they usually don't impact one's ability to function in daily life as much as some other conditions do.

Type 1 diabetes—most often diagnosed in kids—can be associated with some cognitive problems too. Slower speed of processing information and weaker executive functioning skills are the issues most often seen in those with type 1 diabetes, particularly in kids diagnosed with diabetes prior to age 7. That being said, cognitive changes in this form of diabetes are usually milder than those seen in people diagnosed with diabetes later in life.

Perhaps you're wondering how diabetes affects the brain. In other words, why do we see cognitive changes in diabetics? Scientists believe that these changes occur in a few different ways. Both hypoglycemia and hyperglycemia (low and high levels of glucose in the blood, respectively) can stress the blood vessels of the brain. Particular damage to the brain can be caused by extended periods of hyperglycemia or by frequent and extreme swings in blood sugar levels. Single episodes of hypoglycemia or hyperglycemia can also lead to cognitive problems, although these changes don't tend to last as long. In addition, some brain regions can be smaller in diabetics, particularly the hippocampus and the frontal and temporal lobes of the cerebral cortex. There's also evidence of weaker connections between different brain structures, which can result in slower processing speed.

Notably, diabetes is a risk factor for dementia, particularly if diagnosed in midlife. However, it's important to keep in mind that not all dementias are created equal. Diabetes is linked somewhat to Alzheimer's disease—the most common form of dementia—but is more associated with *vascular dementia*. This form of dementia can be caused by chronic damage to the brain's blood vessels, or by multiple small strokes, called *microinfarcts*. Diabetes often occurs alongside other medical problems such as high blood pressure and obesity, which are associated with their own negative effects on the brain. We'll come back to this point shortly.

A few chapters back, we discussed the importance of the Mediterranean diet for a brain-healthy lifestyle. There's some related research indicating that adhering to the MeDi might also prevent type 2 diabetes. And gaining better control over blood sugar levels is linked to greater overall brain size and improved cognition, especially regarding working memory. More generally, physical activity is one of the best ways to reduce the impact of diabetes on the body and the brain. All of the benefits of exercise we covered earlier in the book apply here too. There's the added benefit of improving general health with increased physical fitness, even at relatively low levels.

High Blood Pressure and Obesity

High blood pressure—also known as hypertension—is fairly common and becomes increasingly so as we age. In fact, a recent survey found that about a third of U.S. adults have high blood pressure (a reading of at least 140/90 systolic/diastolic pressure, if you're wondering), and the amount of people with this condition hasn't really changed for at least 15 years. It's also quite common among African American men and women. And from age 60 and up, most people (more than 60%) are hypertensive.

Part of why I'm addressing this topic here is that high blood pressure can not only lead to heart attacks and other cardiovascular problems, but can also reduce brain functioning. Hypertension affects the ability of blood vessels to efficiently circulate blood throughout the brain and also breaks down the brain's white matter—the connective fibers that link one part of the brain to another. One clear brain-related risk associated with hypertension is stroke, although it also has been linked to mild cognitive impairment, dementia, and other cognitive difficulties.

Hypertension is known to diminish multiple cognitive skills, with memory being particularly affected. Executive functions and language abilities can be impacted too. Multiple studies have also shown that having high blood pressure, including in middle age, can increase the chance of cognitive impairment down the road. Some recent research found that hypertension was linked to a *65% increased risk* of dementia for women. There's also evidence that midlife high blood pressure can eventually lead to dementia in men, although successfully reducing blood pressure can minimize the risk of cognitive problems. Overall, we can think of blood pressure as a modifiable lifestyle factor tied to brain-related and general health, and the sooner it can be scaled back to normal levels, the better.

One recent study specifically looked at how exercise affected cognition in people with cardiovascular problems, most of whom had high blood pressure. At the beginning of the study, these folks were generally sedentary; they were exercising no more than twice per week for less than half an hour. Then, for the next 6 months, they were asked to exercise three times per week by walking or cycling for 35 minutes per session. They were also educated about the DASH diet. As we discussed in Chapter 8, this diet is similar to the Mediterranean diet and emphasizes reduced dietary sodium.

For those of you with hypertension, this study offers good news: people who exercised showed significant improvements in executive functioning skills such as flexible thinking and working memory. Eating a DASH-style diet boosted the same skills even more, though only in the people who also exercised. Keep in mind that some earlier research has found specific cognitive benefits from the DASH diet independent of other factors like exercise, so even making brain-healthy dietary changes in isolation can be a good move. Perhaps it goes without saying that even if you have some medical concerns, exercise and dietary changes can really make a difference in how well your brain works.

Another related topic is obesity. Obesity (defined as a body mass index, or BMI, of 30+) is a major public health problem that is not going away. At this point, more than one-third of U.S. adults are obese, and significant weight problems are particularly common in middle age (40% of adults struggle in this regard). Folks who are overweight tend to have high blood pressure, so what we reviewed earlier certainly applies to weight challenges too. But there's another layer to consider: obesity is associated with brain changes independent of other factors. Indeed, having no health issues other than being overweight is linked to less brain volume in certain areas. For example, regions such as the frontal lobes and hippocampus are known to be smaller in those struggling with their weight.

Being overweight or obese can also affect your thinking skills, particularly executive functioning. Some research has found that being overweight can interfere with your ability to make decisions, plan, and think flexibly. The research is somewhat mixed, meaning that cognitive problems won't necessarily be experienced by everyone with weight concerns, but there is a risk of these types of lapses.

More generally, obesity has a disconcerting association with mild cognitive impairment and Alzheimer's disease. As with diabetes, being obese in midlife significantly increases one's chances of cognitive problems many years down the road. Multiple studies following thousands of people over time have demonstrated a connection between obesity and dementia. Adding insult to injury, high total cholesterol levels—common in obesity—also make one more vulnerable to dementia, particularly if those levels are elevated during middle age.

Fortunately, there are some positive or protective factors to keep in mind with obesity and being overweight. First off, if you're struggling with weight but are also physically fit, you're less likely to have major medical problems. Some science indicates that becoming more physically active may be more important for your health than just shedding weight. There's also evidence that reducing your weight can lead to improved thinking skills, including better memory. Harking back to our chapter on nutrition, it's important to note that a Mediterranean-style diet can help with weight reduction and lower "bad" cholesterol levels. These changes are great for overall health and brain health too.

Is Your Brain Going Up in Smoke?

If you're a smoker, you've probably heard from a number of people that you should quit. I would certainly say the same thing. But you also know that it's one of the toughest things *to* quit. Many people spend years going cold turkey, starting up again, and continuing the cycle over and over. I see this pattern frequently with my patients, and it's testament to how addictive nicotine is. It also clarifies how triggers or cues in our environment (like smelling smoke or being with other smokers) make it that much harder to kick the habit. While there have been recent calls to reduce nicotine levels in cigarettes to potentially decrease the number of people who get hooked, smoking will undoubtedly remain a major public health concern for many years to come.

If you're looking for additional motivation to give up smoking, here it is: smoking is really bad *for the brain*. As a neuropsychologist, I'm familiar with lots of things that negatively affect the brain—brain injury, dementia, multiple sclerosis, and stroke, to name a few—but the field of neuropsychology hasn't focused much on smoking as a cognitive culprit until recently. This simply wasn't information I learned during my training years ago. However, when we look at the science of smoking and the brain, there are plenty of reasons to raise the alarm about the dangers of this habit on brain health.

Smoking appears to affect the brain on levels large and small. Smokers have been found to experience global atrophy of the brain—overall brain shrinkage—and reduced size of multiple regions including the frontal, temporal, and occipital lobes. There tend to be small lesions in smokers' white matter: the critically important brain tissue that allows for efficient transmission of signals throughout the brain. There's also evidence for a dose–response relationship between smoking and brain functioning; in other words, the longer someone smokes, the more damage the brain sustains.

In terms of specific cognitive abilities, smoking can impair our efforts to learn and remember new information we hear or see—verbal and nonverbal memory—and how quickly we think and reason. Smokers also show worse mental flexibility and working memory. These types of problems are seen in smokers of all ages, anywhere from people in their teens to adults in their sixties and beyond. Multiple studies have also shown that smokers' thinking skills decline faster over time than those of non-smokers.

Experts agree that as a strategy to prevent different forms of dementia, quitting smoking definitely counts. For example, one large study followed nearly 9,000 people in their early forties for about 25 years. The goal of the study was to determine what sorts of factors in midlife might predict a diagnosis of dementia many years later. We've already covered some of the things that were linked to dementia in this study: hypertension, diabetes, and high cholesterol. Smoking was another lifestyle choice that ramped up dementia risk—by 26%. Other scientists have proposed that *millions* of individuals worldwide could have potentially avoided Alzheimer's disease by not smoking.

Fortunately, if you quit smoking or are in the process of doing so, keep this in mind: smoking cessation is tied to stronger cognitive skills. The science indicates that kicking the habit can result in memory and executive function gains over time, probably within a few years. After about 10 years of not smoking, ex-smokers show expected age-related cognitive changes at about the same rate as people who have never smoked. So giving up cigarettes after being a long-term smoker has compelling benefits on multiple levels.

I'll say it again: what we do in middle age—the types of activities we engage in, and the choices we make about diet, managing our medical problems, and not smoking—has significant implications for our brain and general health many decades in the future.

THE BOTTOM LINE

Here are a few key points related to medical conditions, smoking, and brain health:

- Diabetes—type 1 or type 2—is associated with multiple cognitive difficulties, including problems with memory, processing speed, and executive functioning.
- Diabetes can also increase the risk of developing dementia.
- Eating a Mediterranean-style diet and exercising can prevent diabetes; both lifestyle choices can also reduce the impact of diabetes on the brain.
- Hypertension has been linked to mild cognitive impairment, dementia, and other cognitive challenges.
- Reducing blood pressure through exercise and diets such as the DASH diet can improve general health and brain health.
- Being overweight or obese can lead to mild cognitive difficulties, especially regarding the executive functions.

- Reducing weight through diet or exercise can improve brain health.
- Smoking can diminish the size of multiple brain regions and impair memory, executive functioning, and processing speed; it also increases the chances of developing dementia.
- People who stop smoking show improvement in multiple cognitive skills over time.

THE BRASS TACKS:
PERSONAL STRATEGIC PLANNING TO
BETTER MANAGE MY MEDICAL CONDITIONS
OR TO QUIT SMOKING (use the items below for
either issue)

Topics mentioned in this chapter that I'm struggling to manage better: _____

_____

_____

Factors that get in the way of me improving my medical issues: _____

_____

_____

Something I listed above that I could change to improve my medical issues: _____

_____

_____

Top two things I could try to improve my medical issues:

1. _____

_____

2. _____

_____

Strategies that I can use to improve #1: _____

_____

_____

Strategies that I can use to improve #2: _____

_____

_____

Small steps I can take to improve my medical issues (even a little bit more) this week: _____

_____

_____

Small steps I can take to improve my medical issues (even a little bit more) this month: _____

_____

_____

Goals I have for myself over the next 3 months related to managing my medical issues: _____

_____

_____

Goals I have for myself over the next 6 months related to managing my medical issues: _____

_____

_____

Things I've learned from this chapter that could help me improve my medical issues: _____

_____

_____

_____

How managing my medical issues better is consistent with my current values: _____

_____

_____

_____

PART IV

Moving Forward: Translating Inspiration Into Action

12

Locking in Brain-Healthy Lifestyle Changes

WE'VE NOW COVERED A NUMBER OF IMPORTANT topics related to brain health, and hopefully you've begun to consider these more often in your daily life. Maybe you've made progress with exercise, nutrition, mental activity, sleep hygiene, stress management, or another area. You may have had some success using the worksheets at the end of earlier chapters to help move you in the direction you'd like to go. But change is a long and meandering process. The classic "two steps forward, one step back" is, well, a classic saying for a reason. Initial excitement and interest in making a change can fade, not unlike a New Year's resolution, particularly when something gets in the way early on. It would be nice to think that we can just will ourselves to change our behavior, but unfortunately, this usually isn't how it works. It can really be a hard slog to wire in a new habit or lifestyle change. There are many factors that can help or harm this process, which include things that you might not expect. Even our beliefs about how change occurs can positively or negatively affect our lifestyle goals.

In this chapter, we'll review the science of habit change in more detail while considering topics we've covered earlier in the book. If you've been having trouble moving forward with a new change, I hope that ideas here will make it easier to forge ahead in the interest of a healthier brain. And it may go without saying that our discussion here relates to the "E" of the C.A.P.E. model: *education about the brain* in the context of creating brain-healthy habits.

Let's first consider a habit of sorts that most of us can relate to: learning to drive a car. For most of us, this occurs in the teenage years and involves a few people who facilitate the process: a parent, an older sibling, a driving instructor, maybe others. While the desire to drive is usually high, translating that desire into action is no small task. Hours and hours of time and frustration are devoted to learning how to use the accelerator and brakes, steering wheel, turn signals, and so on. This is very effortful and cognitively demanding, but after months of effort, the process becomes fairly automatic. If you drove a car today, you probably didn't think about many if any of the driving-related skills you developed years ago, and were likely concentrating on higher-order things (like finding a good song on the radio or deciding whether ordering take-out is the best plan for dinner tonight). As we'll see, getting better at driving actually has some important parallels with lifestyle changes we've discussed throughout the book.

THE BACKGROUND SCIENCE
Brain-Healthy Lifestyle Changes
Don't Happen Overnight

If you're struggling to get started with a new brain-boosting activity—or find that managing the obstacles that get in the way is really hard—don't worry, you're not alone. About 50% of people who intend to change their behavior fail to do so. The fact that you're reading this chapter, and this book, indicates that you're interested in the topic and motivated to learn new actionable strategies. Let's consider ways that we can join the 50% of people who *do* change their behavior in a positive direction.

You may be wondering how long will it take for new lifestyle tweaks to become part of your routine over the long haul. What do we know about the time it takes to establish a new habit? There's a study that provides some interesting insights here. A group of young adults was asked to consider a type of behavior they wanted to add to their lives, such as exercising, following a healthier diet, or meditating. They were then instructed to choose a behavior that followed a reminder, or cue, every day, and this cue could only occur once per day (such as trying a new behavior every day after breakfast). They had to submit a daily report to the researchers indicating whether they'd actually engaged in whatever habit they wanted to incorporate.

The study participants were followed for about 3 months. The scientists specifically wanted to understand how quickly new habits became automatic; that is, whether people spontaneously engaged in a habit after a daily event, such as a meal. As is the case in the real world, many people did not establish automatic behaviors by the time the study was completed. About half of the participants fell into this group. However, the other half was different: their new habits became consistent by 12 weeks, and sometimes quite a bit sooner. *The average time it took to lock in a habit was 66 days.* It was a bit easier to adopt changes in diet (an average of 65 days) than to add in an exercise habit (91 days). The study also found that missing one day while trying to build a new habit wasn't a big deal. But other research has shown that missing more time than that, particularly in the early stages of a new activity, can effectively wipe out your gains and send you back to square one.

One interesting study specifically looked at how long it takes to develop a new exercise routine. Researchers followed a group of 94 people over the course of a few months, and the scientists tried to determine at what point people exercised in a habitual way—this was defined as how often the study participants went to the gym at least weekly (the researchers monitored this by seeing how often people swiped their gym membership cards at the gym entrance). It turned out that the tipping point for establishing an exercise habit was right about 5 weeks: the more often people went to the gym throughout that window, the more likely they would maintain the habit in the long run. Conversely, if people slacked off too much in the first 5 weeks—especially if they skipped at least a week—their efforts to exercise were probably doomed. Sticking with a lifestyle change over the course of time, and quickly correcting the inevitable setbacks, is a healthy and realistic way to move forward with a better brain.

Ways We Think About Developing Habits

When we consider how habits are formed, research points to four key steps. First, we need to decide that it's time to make some sort of a lifestyle change. Perhaps it's exercising more, eating less junk food, or learning to play a musical instrument. Second comes the decision to actually do something related to this change, such as starting an exercise routine or clearing out the cookies and chips from your pantry. This is a challenging step, described as the *intention–behavior gap*; we all have ideas on how to improve our lives, but changing our behaviors to align with our plans tends to be pretty difficult. As we discussed earlier, half of those intending to incorporate a new health-oriented habit—like exercising or even getting screened for cancer—fail to do so. It can certainly be an uphill battle to build a new lifestyle change into your life.

Making it to the third step of habit formation is difficult; this particularly critical step involves repeating our new habit over and over again. Doing something just once or twice is recipe for a quick return to your personal status quo—repetition is critical to lock in any lifestyle habit.

The final step to establish a habit is to repeat something

enough that it becomes automatic. This might translate into a regular walk or workout at the gym every Tuesday and Thursday after breakfast, or seeking out carrots instead of Oreos when you start craving a mid-afternoon snack. From a brain-based standpoint, something becomes habitual when you no longer have to think deliberately about doing it (dominion of the frontal lobes) and instead establish an effective, automatic routine (governed by some regions below the cerebral cortex, including the basal ganglia).

I play guitar, and sometimes I hear a song that I'd like to learn. This happens enough that I've created a list of songs that I hope to work on at some point. Jumping from my aspirational list to actually starting to learn a song—my own intention–behavior gap—takes some effort. I need to look for an instructional video on YouTube, find guitar tablature in a music shop or online, or try to figure out the song on my own (the latter usually being the least efficient strategy).

Once I've committed to a certain song and have found instructional material I can use to help me learn it, I need to practice it over and over, dozens if not hundreds of times. Unless I really like the song, or contain my frustration just enough while struggling with the intricacies of how to play certain notes or combinations of notes, I'm sunk. Eventually, the song will become automatic, but it takes a lot of time and effort (and serious patience). So, for what it's worth, I can directly relate to the importance of completing all four steps of habit formation. Everyone has the potential for both successes and missed opportunities in this regard.

Of course, our negative habits may have formed in a similar way. Routinely eating potato chips or other unhealthy snacks while watching a sports game, favorite TV show, or streaming series began as something novel and then became habitual. Good habits are great to hold on to; bad habits are understandably hard to kick. We'll come back to this point later in the chapter.

One way to increase the chances of successfully incorporating a new lifestyle change is to have a built-in reminder, or cue. This could be a reminder that occurs at a certain time of the day, although an even better cue is one that is linked to an event. That way, you're not complicating things by relying on time. Perhaps a meal or a weekly meeting can serve as a reminder: these are consistent, concrete events, which tend to be particularly useful in cueing us to do something. Let's say you're hoping to read more often; the reminder of seeing the newspaper on your driveway in the morning is a simple but effective cue to start one's day. Exercising before a meal or after a regularly scheduled meeting could work the same way (especially if it tends to be a meeting that ramps up stress that needs to be burned off later).

Ben was a client of mine who became interested in meditation as a way to manage his stress. He was also very interested to learn about the brain-related benefits of mindfulness (similar to what we covered in Chapter 10), although his initial efforts were slow going. He had a meditation app on his phone that he liked, but he was having trouble using the app consistently. We discussed potential ways to build meditation into his life with a cue such as a specific meal. He decided that lunchtime was a perfect reminder for him, and he started doing a 5-minute meditation exercise right before he ate lunch. This actually ended up serving two purposes: he had a consistent event that he wouldn't forget as a reminder—he never skipped lunch—and he began eating more slowly and mindfully as a function of being in a more relaxed state after meditating.

Another thing to mention: While it's unclear whether some sort of tangible reward you give yourself (like a fancy coffee or sweet snack) can help or harm your ability to create a new habit, the science really emphasizes the value of *internal rewards* when pursuing a goal. Being personally motivated to engage in a new activity is particularly powerful. Along these lines, earlier in the book we discussed the flow state—the experience we have while engaging in an activity that is challenging but also enjoyable and stimulating. Being in a flow state is internally rewarding, and the activities that get us there are sure to motivate us to try them again. In a related vein, enjoying a new activity clearly increases the chances of us continuing to do it: this is a common finding in positive psychology research.

Take a moment to reflect: What's something you do well? Perhaps a hobby, a sport, or a work-related activity you excel at? How did you develop your skills in this area, and how long did it take? A strategy or process that worked in the past can be an ally of sorts as you plot out a new lifestyle change. There might be a piece of what worked before that could be valuable (maybe even really valuable) for you now.

Keep An Eye on What You're Doing, and Follow a Plan

One of the most effective ways of changing our behavior is monitoring it. Sounds simple, and it can be, but consistently keeping track of how much we're exercising, socializing, eating nutritiously, and so on really matters. Throughout the book, you've hopefully been doing this. My goal has been to give you related tools—in the form of self-monitoring worksheets—to kick-start your desired changes. For any lifestyle tweak we hope to make, it's imperative to understand what our baseline is for that behavior, what our plan is for moving forward, and how to deal with potential barriers that can potentially get in the way of our goals.

Plenty of research supports the value of monitoring our behavior when we want to make a change. One study looked at factors linked to how well people were able to improve their diets and build in an exercise routine. This was a massive study—over 40,000 people across dozens of smaller studies—and focused on 26 different strategies people can use to positively modify their lifestyle choices. Across all behavior-change techniques, one was head and shoulders above the rest: *self-monitoring*. Simply put, in order to make a change, we need to know what we're currently doing by keeping track of our behaviors.

In a similar vein, having a specific plan of attack related to changing our behavior—one that we can revise as needed—is also critical. Being too optimistic about changing our behavior can be just as problematic as being a negative Nancy. We need to find a happy medium between having a goal and acknowledging potential roadblocks on the way to our goal. Making the steps of our goal concrete and well-defined, rather than aspirational and vague, propels us forward and helps us anticipate inevitable challenges.

The study I mentioned above found that beyond monitoring our behavior, things like setting goals for how we'll change our behaviors and reviewing those goals periodically were also important to improve lifestyle choices (and, we can safely conclude, overall wellness). And don't be afraid to tell others what you're working on: research shows that we're better at achieving our goals when we've let others know what they are. This serves a related purpose, which is having support from people in your life with what you're taking on. They're more likely to provide encouragement and advice and may even steer you away from problematic distractions.

Another powerful strategy is to physically record how we're doing with our goals. Writing them down on a list or a sticky note or using an app on a smartphone or other device increases the chances of accomplishing what we set out to do. Along these lines, you may have heard of SMART goals.

This acronym stands for five useful reminders that define what a goal should look like:

- Specific
- Measurable
- Attainable
- Relevant
- Time-based

This is a nice framework for any goal, and we can use this here for goals you may have related to brain health. Let's say you've been wanting to shift your diet so that your meals more consistently include foods from the brain-boosting Mediterranean diet. You could use the SMART acronym like this:

- *Specific*: I'll have a meal with fish and green leafy vegetables at least once a week.
- *Measurable*: I'll monitor my fish and veggie consumption in a journal that will stay in the kitchen.
- *Attainable*: I'll start my goal by eating in this way once a week, which is a shift for me but one that I can make happen.
- *Relevant*: I'm interested in improving my brain health, and this is one way to do it.
- *Time-based*: I'll make this dietary change for a month and will reassess my goal and any tweaks I might want to make after that.

Or, how about trying to exercise more consistently:

- *Specific*: I'll go on a brisk 30-minute walk at lunch on Tuesday and Thursday over the next month.
- *Measurable*: I'll keep track of my exercise using a notes app on my smartphone.
- *Attainable*: I'm usually reading or surfing the Internet during the lunch hour, so carving out a few 30-minute windows to exercise is doable.
- *Relevant*: I know that exercise is really good for my brain, so this is a meaningful goal for me.
- *Time-based*: I'll try this exercise routine for the next month and reevaluate at that point.

A related issue is managing bad habits that can get in the way of establishing positive, healthy habits. Let's say you're trying to work on sleeping 7 to 8 hours per night, and you have trouble doing this because you're a big fan of late-night comedy shows. While laughing is certainly great medicine, the benefits of getting a good night of sleep far outweigh watching a late program live. As we talked about earlier, cues or reminders in our environment can help or hurt the process of forming positive habits. In this case, seeing the TV remote can cue us to follow two paths (Figure 12.1).

Research provides some important insights here too. What's referred to as *vigilant monitoring*—essentially being on the lookout for cues that prompt bad habits, like grabbing the TV remote and pushing the power button when

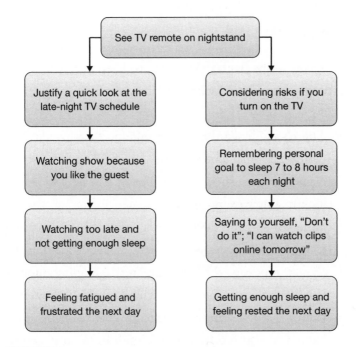

FIGURE 12.1

you're about to go to sleep—is a particularly effective way to manage temptations that throw you off course. In this case, you could say to yourself, "Don't do it" or "I know what could happen here if I pick up that remote." More generally, distracting yourself from a bad habit by doing something else, or leaving the room or setting where you're tempted to do something you'll regret, can help you stick with the positive change you're trying to maintain.

THE BOTTOM LINE

Here are a few tips from the chapter to keep in mind as you incorporate brain-healthy habits into your life:

- There's evidence that it can take 66 or more days to firmly establish a new habit.
- Some research shows that we need at least 5 weeks to lock in a new exercise routine.
- Four key steps to developing a new habit are deciding to make a change, taking action to begin making the change, repeating the behavior, and developing automaticity (engaging in the habit without thinking about it).
- Having a consistent reminder, or cue, to help kick a habit into gear is critical to maintaining (and strengthening) a habit over time.
- Internal satisfaction is better than external rewards when trying to incorporate a new brain-healthy habit.
- Monitoring your current behavior is one of the most important steps toward making a change in your lifestyle.
- Devise a detailed plan when starting a new lifestyle behavior. Creating a SMART plan (specific, measurable, attainable, relevant, time-based) can be particularly useful, especially if it's written down or recorded another way (such as on a smartphone).
- Be on the lookout for temptations and distractions that can throw you off course while building in a new lifestyle change or that lead you to engage in a negative habit.

THE BRASS TACKS:
PERSONAL STRATEGIC PLANNING TO
LOCK IN BRAIN-HEALTHY CHANGES

Primary activity or behavior I'm trying to work into my routine: _____

_____

_____

Successes I've had so far in incorporating this activity:

_____

_____

_____

Challenges or setbacks I've had so far in incorporating this activity: _____

_____

_____

The part of the four key steps to establishing a habit that I've had trouble with: _____

_____

_____

Reminders, or cues, that are helping me stay on track (or ones I can use in the future): _____

_____

_____

What I learned in the past while developing a new habit or skill that could be relevant now: _____

_____

_____

_____

A SMART goal I can make to help me lock in my brain-healthy lifestyle change:

Specific: _____

_____

Measurable: _____

_____

Attainable: _____

_____

Realistic: _____

_____

Time-based: _____

_____

Changes I plan to make based on what I've read in this chapter: _____

_____

_____

_____

How these changes are consistent with my current values:

_____

_____

_____

_____

Now, go back to the end of Chapter 1 and re-rate yourself
on the lifestyle questions at the end of the chapter. What
changes have you made compared to how you rated yourself
before? What are you still working on? _____

_____

_____

_____

_____

_____

An Executive Summary of Bottom Lines for Brain Health

IN THE SPIRIT OF OUR BOTTOM-LINE SUMMARIES throughout the book, here's a final executive summary of some of the key points related to improving your brain health:

The C.A.P.E. Model Summarizes Four Key Domains of Brain Health

- Cognitive strategies
- Activity engagement
- Prevention of cognitive problems
- Education about the brain

Cognitive Strategies

- Try to find a balance between using internal (self-generated) and external (something physical, like a calendar or sticky notes) strategies to help you remember and manage daily tasks.

- To promote your attention, verbalize or "talk yourself through" tasks.

- To enhance your memory for new things, use repetition, add personal associations, draw what you're trying to remember, and put information into an easily remembered "package" such as an acronym or a story.

- Keep task lists brief, and try to complete one task at a time before moving onto something else.

- If you're struggling to figure out a daily problem, take a mental step back, take some deep breaths, and ask yourself if there are other options you might not have considered.

- When taking on a new task, increase the chances of getting into a flow state: prepare well before you start, make sure you have all the resources you need, and try to maintain a positive and engaged attitude.

Exercise and the Brain

- Any amount or type of exercise is good for the brain, although most related research has looked at the brain-boosting effects of casual or brisk walking.

- Physical fitness at any point in life, but particularly in midlife, decreases the chance of developing Alzheimer's disease.

- Even low levels of physical activity can reduce the risk of cardiovascular and other health problems.
- Exercising at least 10 to 15 minutes per day leads to brain and cognitive benefits; 20 to 30 minutes per day is even better.
- Moderately intense exercise (a 5 to 6 rating on a 0 to 10 scale of minimum to maximum exertion) is especially beneficial for brain health and cognitive abilities like executive functioning.
- Adding a social component to exercise might help your brain more than exercising alone, and may help you stick with an exercise routine.

Socializing and the Brain

- Socializing with others on a regular basis is good for emotional *and* brain health.
- Social interactions lasting at least 10 minutes have stronger brain-based benefits than shorter ones; think of getting consistent social "doses" that last at least this long.
- The larger your social network, the better your brain tends to work, and the lower your risk of dementia.
- Feeling supported by others is emotionally enriching *and* has brain-related benefits.
- Negative social encounters and loneliness are detrimental to the brain and cognitive abilities.
- Volunteering in the community has a great side effect: improved brain health.

Mental Activities and the Brain

- Being involved in mentally stimulating hobbies such as reading, playing board games, photography, doing crossword puzzles, playing a musical instrument, or doing crafts is really positive for brain health.
- Engaging in hobbies for an hour or more per day is best for the brain.
- Participating in hobbies in midlife could protect you from developing dementia in later life.
- Try to be involved with more than one hobby or leisure activity; one is good, two or more are better for cognitive skills and brain health.
- Working in a stimulating job, especially if you manage other people, seems to have protective effects on the brain.
- So-called brain-training games have not consistently been found to benefit brain health in daily life, even if your performance on specific games tends to improve.

Nutrition and the Brain

- Many studies support the Mediterranean diet (MeDi) as a great brain-healthy nutritional style that reduces the risk of cognitive decline and dementia.
- A slightly altered version of the MeDi, the MIND diet, emphasizes berries and leafy and cruciferous vegetables, and might be even better for the brain.
- A Western-style diet, including high saturated fat,

red meat, and processed food, is unhealthy for the brain and cognition.

- Omega-3 fatty acids, particularly when consumed through your diet, do many positive things for brain and cognitive functioning.
- Specific foods like fish, nuts, olive oil, berries, and vegetables have been linked to better brain health.
- Existing science does not support taking over-the-counter nutritional supplements to improve brain functioning.

Sleep and the Brain

- Seven to eight hours per night is the "sweet spot" for general and brain-related wellness.
- Sleeping less than 6 hours per night, or more than 9 hours per night, can be associated with cognitive problems, especially if done across consecutive nights.
- Being mindful of sleep hygiene—avoiding caffeine later in the day, avoiding TV or other screen watching in bed, and having consistent sleep and wake times—can help promote more satisfying sleep.
- Afternoon naps of less than 30 minutes can temporarily enhance multiple cognitive abilities, including how well we learn and remember new information.
- Sleep apnea can reduce attention, processing speed, memory, and executive functioning, but use of a CPAP device can help cognitive skills improve.

- High school students who start classes at 8:30 AM or later—and are able to sleep more as a result—have better cognitive, emotional, and behavioral health.

Mellowing the Stressed Brain

- Stress is a very subjective experience, in that what's stressful for one person can be interesting or joyful for someone else.
- Stress can negatively affect the hippocampus and frontal lobes, leading to reduced memory and executive functioning skills.
- Mindfulness meditation strategies and yoga can improve cognitive abilities and increase the size of multiple brain regions.
- Gratitude exercises, such as writing down things you're grateful for a few times per week, can reduce stress and bring down your blood pressure.
- Affirming values that are important to you can be an effective stress-reduction technique.
- Exercise can reduce stress and improve your mood, both in the moment and over time.

Effects of Medical Problems and Smoking on the Brain

- Diabetes can lead to multiple cognitive problems, particularly as related to memory, processing speed, and executive functioning.
- High blood pressure and obesity are also linked to cognitive difficulties.

- Diabetes, hypertension, and obesity are risk factors for different types of dementia including Alzheimer's disease.

- Exercise, a Mediterranean-style diet, and the DASH diet can all reduce the effects of medical problems on the brain.

- Smoking has been linked to reduced brain size, cognitive deficits, and dementia.

- People who quit smoking can experience improvement in their thinking skills, although it may take a few years for this to happen.

Locking in Brain-Healthy Lifestyle Changes

- Establishing a new habit or lifestyle change takes time. Research shows that it takes at least 5 weeks for exercise habits to become routine; habits in general have been found to take about 66 days to get locked in.

- After deciding to adopt a new brain-healthy change and starting to make the change, lots of repetition of the behavior is needed to make it automatic.

- Monitoring your current behavior is a critically important step toward making a change in your lifestyle.

- Reminders, or cues (like exercising before or after a specific meal every day), can help establish a new habit and maintain it over time.

- Create a detailed, written plan for how you're going to move forward to improve your brain health. One option is to make a SMART goal: one that is specific, measurable, attainable, relevant, and time-based.

- Be mindful of distractions that can get in the way of establishing a new habit, and develop strategies to help you stay focused on your goal.

ACKNOWLEDGMENTS

Writing a book over the course of multiple years involved the direct and indirect support of many people. I am immensely grateful to all of them.

First, I greatly appreciate Peter Arnett, Heather Wishart, Jennifer Randolph, Lauren Strober, Chris Higginson, Maureen Schmitter-Edgecombe, Naomi Chaytor, Robert Roth, Patricia Pimental, Ben Hill, Maureen O'Connor, Malissa Kraft, Bruce Levine, Amanda Rabinowitz, Stephen Aita, Dede Ukueberuwa, Gray Vargas, Ronald Ruff, Ruben Echemendia, Michelle Braun, Robert Ferguson, Bill Gunn, Justin Miller, Sarah Banks, and other colleagues and friends for our stimulating discussions and collaborative projects related to brain health, resilience, and related topics.

Many thanks to Dawn Huebner for her encouragement and sage advice on translating professional content for a general audience.

Thanks also to Robert Emmons for introducing me to the gratitude-neuroscience literature.

I feel blessed to have generous friends and colleagues who have graciously read portions of the book and provided helpful suggestions. I thank you all: Travis Lovejoy, Paul Wager, Vicky Drucker, Kate St. James, Michael Campos, Paul Kwon, Joanne Berns, Paul Gallagher, Jane Torpie, and Peter Thorne.

Thanks to friends Bruce Levine and Tony Abbate, both of whom help support my brain health through physical and social engagement as we battle it out on the racquetball and tennis courts.

I am also grateful to my Osher@Dartmouth students over the years who have further inspired my interest in promoting brain health and desire to communicate related ideas into communities near and far.

Thanks to Angelina Lionetta for her helpful suggestion to include a list of book club questions for readers.

I am deeply indebted to my editor, Deborah Malmud, for her interest in and enthusiasm for this book project, and for her instrumental suggestions and support throughout the process. Thanks also to Sara McBride, Mariah Eppes, Kevin Olsen, Megan Bedell, Nicholas Fuenzalida, and others at W. W. Norton for their administrative and logistical assistance.

A special note of gratitude to my wonderful wife, Jen, for her encouragement, scientific consultation, and support throughout this journey.

This book is lovingly dedicated to my cognitively robust, multitalented, emotionally intelligent, and overall amazing daughter, Kaia.

BOOK CLUB QUESTIONS

1. What brain health topic was most interesting for you?
2. What research described in the book was most unexpected?
3. How much did you know about the brain and neuroscience before reading this book?
4. What did you think of the evidence related to how activities affect brain health? Was the evidence more compelling for any specific activity?
5. What were the top two or three things you learned from the book that you didn't know before?
6. How much did you use the "Brass Tacks" sections to help promote new changes?
7. How do you plan to use what you learned from the book in the future?
8. Would you want to read another book like this in the future?
9. Did this book make you want to learn more about the brain and neuroscience?

For Each Chapter

1. What were one or two takeaways from this chapter that you'd like to incorporate into your life?

2. What did you learn in this chapter that was surprising or unexpected?

3. What did you hope to learn more about in this chapter?

4. How useful was the worksheet at the end of the chapter?

The "Science" in Neuroscience

A core foundation of this book is neuroscience research. While *neuroscience* as a term sounds futuristic and sexy, the science in neuroscience certainly can have its flaws. If we are to rely on neuroscience research findings, we need to be able to gauge whether the science has been done well.

In many of the studies discussed in this book, researchers have sought to understand one factor among many that can potentially answer a scientific question. For example, a study that aims to determine whether social activity is good for the brain will measure how socially engaged someone is and will also assess brain functioning, usually with neuropsychological tests or with brain-imaging techniques. All of these variables can be measured in multiple ways, which can affect what the study ultimately reveals. So, social activity could be assessed by gauging how much time someone socializes each day, how many people that individual sees on a regular basis, that individual's level of social support, and so on.

Scientists need to demonstrate that a study's findings accurately answer the question being asked, and ensure that there isn't something else going on that mucks up the data. So, for research looking at the effects of social engagement on cognitive skills, it would be important to account for or *control for* other factors. Some of these might include age (socializing could affect memory more in older adults than younger adults), education (college graduates might reap the cognitive benefits of socializing better than those with less education), or physical activity (people who are more social might also tend to exercise, another factor that has a powerful effect on cognitive skills). Since these other factors, or *confounds*, could partly (if not entirely) explain the study's findings, we need to be able to consider their potential role in what we're trying to understand. There are some sophisticated statistical techniques that allow us to adjust for confounds that could affect study results; suffice it to say that these methods are used by researchers on a regular basis.

Some research examines brain-related effects of an intervention, such as a new exercise program or a dietary change. For these studies, researchers need to create roughly equivalent *treatment* and *control* groups. These groups need to be about the same regarding age, education, gender, and sometimes other factors. If they differ, the ultimate conclusions from the study can be flawed, because differences between the group that got the intervention and the one that didn't could simply reflect differences in how the groups were composed.

For example, it wouldn't make much sense to compare the cognitive effects of an exercise program on a group of people in their thirties (the *treatment* group) relative to a group of people in their fifties who weren't exercising (the *control* group). A much better study design would compare people of similar ages, right? That way, we know that the effects of any sort of lifestyle change are due to the intervention itself rather than factors we're less interested in.

We also need to be mindful of where research is being published. In this day and age, there are many scientific journals in each academic field, some at the top of their game and others at or near the bottom. Publishing findings in a middling journal is easier than getting your results into a well-regarded one, but you can still claim to have published your study in an academic journal. This sometimes legitimizes research that is poorly conducted and fundamentally flawed. Adding insult to injury, lately there has been an uptick in journals that allow researchers to publish their findings merely by paying to do so, with little or no peer review involved (that is, having some of your colleagues look over your study before agreeing to publish it). As much as possible, I have tried to consider and cite research that comes from well-regarded journals in fields such as neuropsychology, other psychology subfields (such as clinical and social psychology), neuroscience, gerontology, neurology, neuroimaging, general and preventative medicine, and epidemiology.

Another important point relates to the size of a study. All studies are not created equal, and we need to be aware of the sample size before we consider drawing broad conclusions about an interesting result. Research described in this book is usually from studies using moderate or large sample sizes, mainly because the more people that have been studied, the more powerful the results tend to be. When possible, I've also tried to comment on findings that have been observed across multiple studies; results from a single, well-conducted study are interesting, but similar findings across a few studies are even more compelling and provide better evidence for a broad phenomenon.

Because much of the research cited in the book examines the effects of lifestyle choices on brain functioning and cognitive skills, we need to understand how cognition is being measured. Some studies, particularly the very large ones, tend to use brief *screening measures* of cognition. There might be a few words to memorize, a quick test of mental calculation, and a few questions about awareness of the day of the week and the date. The advantage to using these cognitive screens is that they can be administered to hundreds of research participants fairly easily. The disadvantage is that screening measures often don't tell us much about how someone's brain is working. While they can indicate that someone with a stroke or dementia has significant cognitive impairment, they are much less effective at detecting mild cognitive problems.

As one example, for many years doctors believed that

most individuals with multiple sclerosis (MS) did not experience meaningful memory or other cognitive decline. This conclusion was based on the common use of a simple and fairly crude cognitive screen that was poor at detecting milder deficits. Once individuals with MS were given more extensive batteries of cognitive tests, problems with skills like information processing speed and memory retrieval became apparent. These observations ushered in a new understanding of cognitive problems in MS, and clarified that up to 50% of MS patients show at least mild memory or other cognitive difficulties. In a related vein, research using comprehensive neuropsychological batteries tends to be more effective at detecting cognitive problems—and cognitive *improvement*—compared to brief screening tests.

Because the focus here is on lifestyle factors that can improve our brain health, we need to know what works and what doesn't. So, as much as possible, I've tried to include research that uses more sophisticated measures of cognitive functioning, which generally give us a better sense of what's going on with the brain.

APPENDIX B

A Brief Review of Neuroimaging Techniques

Before the 1990s, our understanding of the brain mostly came from studying people who had sustained brain injuries. The logic was something like this: if someone had a stroke or brain trauma that involved the frontal lobes of the brain, and this person was now more impulsive and irritable than in the past, then the frontal lobes must be associated with regulating our behavior and emotions. Brain-injury case studies like this contributed important information to how the brain works, but mostly how it can break down.

Now, many studies related to neuroscience use powerful brain scanning, or *neuroimaging*, techniques that allow for an intimate view of the brain in individuals both with and without brain injuries. There are two primary types of neuroimaging. *Structural neuroimaging* allows us to either take a picture of the brain as a whole or look at certain regions (or structures), such as the frontal lobes or the hippocampus.

Sometimes neuroimaging research is focused on answering questions about specific brain structures; for example, is the hippocampus smaller in older adults with mild cognitive impairment compared to those without such impairment?

There are ways to not only visualize certain areas but also to quantify the volume of such areas. Structural brain magnetic resonance imaging (brain MRI) is like using MRI for other purposes, where understanding tissue function and dysfunction is important. Say you've experienced some knee pain after playing tennis or jogging. Your physician might recommend getting an MRI to understand whether you have sustained any underlying cartilage or tendon damage. Similarly, structural brain MRI is used to take a detailed set of pictures of the tissue within your cranium, in other words, your brain! Some types of structural neuroimaging include voxel-based morphometry, which is used to quantify brain volume in specific brain regions, and fluid-attenuated inversion recovery (FLAIR) MRI, which helps researchers quantify the volume of brain lesions in neurological diseases such as multiple sclerosis.

Functional neuroimaging is used to understand how the brain is working while engaging in a certain type of task, such as touching your thumb to each of your fingers (a motor task) or memorizing a list of words (a cognitive task). Most of the neuroscience research we see in popular media uses functional neuroimaging. It is innovative and state-of-the-art, and has immensely improved our understanding of brain functioning in daily life.

The most common form of functional neuroimaging is functional MRI (fMRI), which has been used since the early 1990s. It relies on a straightforward principle: when we engage in a specific activity, the brain regions associated with performance related to the activity become engorged with oxygen-rich blood (what is referred to as *oxygenated* blood). fMRI is able to distinguish between the magnetic properties of oxygenated blood and deoxygenated blood very effectively, and the contrast between the two can ultimately be visualized with specialized computer software. This process results in the images you may have seen online or in major newspapers that clarify what brain regions become active during certain types of tasks. While neuroscience techniques are not perfect, they have helped us move leaps and bounds in our understanding of the brain over the past 25 or so years.

Professionals Whose Services Benefit the Brain

People sometimes wonder which healthcare providers and other professionals use and translate information related to brain health in their work. For example, who does one meet with to discuss brain health principles or brain-related problems?

A clinical neuropsychologist is one of the most knowledgeable professionals in this category. Neuropsychologists are doctors who have earned a PhD or PsyD, generally in clinical psychology, and have completed a postdoctoral fellowship in clinical neuropsychology to develop further expertise related to understanding brain–behavior relationships. They are skilled in helping others modify their behavior in positive ways, diagnosing cognitive disorders (or not diagnosing, as the case may be), and determining cognitive strengths and challenges by using sophisticated neuropsychological tests that measure many cognitive abilities.

More specifically, neuropsychologists assess cognitive skills that are critical for functioning well in daily life, including attention and concentration, executive functions (such as problem solving, organization, and flexible thinking), learning and memory, spatial and perceptual skills, receptive and expressive language, fine motor abilities, and emotional health. They will generally review various medical records to understand someone's history, and conduct an extensive interview to learn about the individual's daily life and challenges. After an evaluation, the neuropsychologist usually reviews findings with the individual and communicates these results to the referring clinician, who might be a neurologist, psychiatrist, neurosurgeon, clinical psychologist, or educator. Some people see a neuropsychologist over time, perhaps every few years, to monitor cognitive skills and consider new treatments as needed.

Neurologists are medial doctors who have completed a residency in neurology. They do extensive interviews, use diagnostic tests like MRI to take pictures of the brain, and diagnose brain-based disorders such as multiple sclerosis or Parkinson's disease. Neurologists and neuropsychologists often work hand in hand to understand and treat those with brain injuries or brain diseases. Neurologists might use cognitive screens that assess memory and other skills very quickly, and they often refer patients to neuropsychologists for a more detailed evaluation of cognitive functioning if there seem to be indications of brain-related changes.

Clinical psychologists are doctoral-level clinicians who

are trained in diagnosing and treating psychological problems such as depression and anxiety. They may collaborate with neuropsychologists to help improve mood and behavior over time in someone with brain-based problems. They employ behavioral strategies including cognitive–behavioral therapy and interpersonal therapy, both of which are grounded in extensive research. Psychiatrists are medical doctors who also diagnose and treat difficulties with mood, but they tend to treat these problems using medications. Psychologists and psychiatrists often collaborate to improve mood using both behavioral and medical treatments.

Another professional whose work serves to improve brain skills is the executive functioning coach. This individual is usually a college graduate and may have a master's degree in education or another area. One of the coach's key roles is to create and reinforce strategies for managing school demands on an ongoing basis. Coaches differ from academic tutors in that they help people develop overarching organizational and other executive skills that ideally improve performance across academic subject areas. Executive functioning coaches work with students of all ages but mostly with children and adolescents.

A coach who works exclusively in work settings or with executives is the executive coach. Executive coaches might help their clients improve certain cognitive abilities, such as time management and planning, or reinforce strategies to enhance interpersonal skills in the workplace. In medical settings, health coaches work alongside physicians and other

clinicians to reinforce healthy behavior changes over time
that can benefit the brain and body.

NOTES

CHAPTER 1: The Four Domains of Brain Health

7 *Even then, over 50% of people remain dementia free*: See M. M. Corrada et al. (2008), Prevalence of dementia after age 90: Results from the 90+ study. *Neurology, 71*, 337–343.

7 *They also show memory abilities that rival those of middle-aged adults*: For an example of "Superagers" research, see T.M. Harrison et al. (2012), Superior memory and higher cortical volumes in unusually successful cognitive aging, *Journal of the International Neuropsychological Society, 18*, 1081–1085.

8 *higher physical fitness in midlife is linked to better brain health 20+ years later*: As one example, see N.L. Spartano et al. (2016), Midlife exercise blood pressure, heart rate, and fitness related to brain volume 2 decades later, *Neurology, 86*, 1–7.

8 *a study a few years ago that found that sedentary individuals in their eighties who began an exercise program*: See Q. Tian et al. (2014), Physical activity predicts microstructural integrity in memory-related networks in very old adults, *Journals of Gerontology: Medical Sciences, 69*, 1284–1290.

CHAPTER 2: How Does Neuroscience Relate to Brain Health?

26 *BDNF has been referred to as the "Miracle-Gro" of the brain*: For an easily digestible discussion of this topic, and a review of some of the earlier research on exercise and the brain, see J. Ratey and E. Hagerman (2008), *Spark: The Revolutionary New Science of Exercise and the Brain*, New York, NY: Little, Brown.

29 *As the title of a recent book on H.M. noted*: To learn more about H.M.'s life and memory difficulties, see S. Corkin (2013), *Permanent*

Present Tense: The Unforgettable Life of the Amnesic Patient, H.M., New York, NY: Basic Books.

33 *every year, approximately 10% of people with MCI "convert" to dementia*: For a detailed review of MCI, see R.C. Petersen (2011), Mild cognitive impairment, *New England Journal of Medicine, 364,* 2227–2234.

33 *an image that helps clarify different possible cognitive "trajectories"*: See C. Hertzog et al. (2009), Enrichment effects on adult cognitive development, *Psychological Science in the Public Interest, 9,* 1–65.

37 *One fascinating example of research that relates to brain plasticity was conducted with taxi drivers*: See E.A. Maguire et al. (2000), Navigation-related structural change in the hippocampi of taxi drivers, *Proceedings of the National Academy of Sciences USA, 97,* 4398–4403.

38 *A related concept is cognitive reserve*: For additional discussion of the cognitive reserve concept, see Y. Stern (Ed.) (2007), *Cognitive Reserve: Theory and Applications.* New York, NY: Taylor & Francis.

39 *In an early study, over 600 nuns agreed to undergo cognitive testing every few years*: For a detailed description of this fascinating study, see D. Snowdon (2002), *Aging with Grace: What the Nun Study Teaches Us about Leading Longer, Healthier, and More Meaningful Lives,* New York, NY: Bantam Books.

40 *The results supported the importance of active cognitive reserve from a social standpoint*: See D.A. Bennett et al. (2006), The effect of social networks on the relation between Alzheimer's disease pathology and level of cognitive function in old people: A longitudinal cohort study, *Lancet Neurology, 5,* 406–412.

CHAPTER 3: The Cognitive Trio That Matters Most: Attention, Memory, and Executive Functions

43 *about half of people report memory problems, and at least a third say that they have trouble finding the right word to use in conversation*: A few public surveys have clarified the prevalence of cognitive complaints in the general population. See A. Singh-Manoux et al. (2014), Subjective cognitive complaints and mortality: Does the type of complaint matter? *Journal of Psychiatric Research, 48,* 73–78; see also W. Mittenberg et al. (1993), Recovery from mild head injury: A treatment manual for patients, *Psychotherapy in Private Practice, 12,* 37–52.

45 A study some colleagues and I did a few years ago revealed that memory
    complaints relate to cognitive abilities other than memory: See J.J. Ran-
    dolph et al. (2001), Metamemory and tested cognitive functioning
    in multiple sclerosis, Clinical Neuropsychologist, 15, 357–368.

45 One study with older adults found that people who were more physically
    fit reported fewer instances of forgetting: See A.N. Szabo et al. (2011),
    Cardiorespiratory fitness, hippocampal volume, and frequency of
    forgetting in older adults, Neuropsychology, 25, 545–553.

45 When recalling a past experience, the peak-end rule states that we tend
    to overvalue the most painful "peak" of an experience: D. Kahneman
    (2011), Thinking, Fast and Slow, New York, NY: Farrar, Straus and
    Giroux.

50 People were asked to indicate how often they typically multitasked with
    media: See E. Ophir et al. (2009), Cognitive control in media mul-
    titaskers, Proceedings of the National Academy of Sciences USA, 106,
    15583–15587.

54 he was forever trapped in the brief period of working memory, being
    unable to lock in almost any new information: H.M. was able to
    remember—outside of his awareness—some motor-oriented infor-
    mation. For example, researchers found that his performance on a
    difficult mirror-drawing task—where he was asked to draw a star
    that he viewed in a mirror image—improved quickly over time,
    and he performed this task well over the course of a few days.
    However, despite his time learning how to do the task and related
    improvement, he was not able to consciously recall having done
    the task before. For a detailed description of H.M.'s life, see S.
    Corkin (2013), Permanent present tense: The unforgettable life of the
    amnesic patient, H.M., New York, NY: Basic Books.

54 Similar to some other forms of memory, working memory can be enhanced:
    See P.J. Olesen et al. (2004), Increased prefrontal and parietal activ-
    ity after training of working memory, Nature Neuroscience, 7, 75–79.

54 one study found that working memory gains can occur when we affirm
    our core values: See C. Logel and G.L. Cohen (2012), The role of the
    self in physical health: Testing the effect of a values-affirmation
    intervention on weight loss, Psychological Science, 23, 53–55.

54 Affirming our values can also help with the process of adopting new hab-
    its: See R. Cooke et al. (2014), Self-affirmation promotes physical
    activity, Journal of Sport & Exercise Psychology, 36, 217–223.

58 This brings us to a related concept discussed by psychologist Daniel Gole-

man, called the emotional hijack: See D. Goleman (2005), Emotional Intelligence: Why it Can Matter More than IQ, New York, NY: Bantam Books.

60 The exercise you just did has been associated with a number of positive outcomes: See C. Logel and G.L. Cohen (2012) and R. Cooke et al. (2014) as noted above; see also E.B. Falk et al. (2015), Self-affirmation alters the brain's response to health messages and subsequent behavior change, Proceedings of the National Academy of Sciences USA, 112, 1977–1982.

CHAPTER 4: What Strategies Make the Most Difference?

64 One is a guy named Chao Lu: For a more detailed description, see Y. Hu and K.A. Ericsson (2012), Memorization and recall of very long lists accounted for within the long-term working memory framework, Cognitive Psychology, 64, 235–266.

65 Some researchers found out about this and decided to pay Buenos Aires a visit: See T.A. Bekinschtein et al. (2008), Strategies of Buenos Aires waiters to enhance memory capacity in a real-life setting, Behavioural Neurology, 20, 65–70.

68 Daniel Kahneman has demonstrated in his research: See D. Kahneman (2011), Thinking, fast and slow. New York, NY: Farrar, Straus, and Giroux.

68 as we know from positive psychology research, it's much easier to develop a positive lifestyle habit: For a detailed discussion of the role of positive emotion on behavior change, see B.L. Fredrickson (2013), Chapter One - Positive emotions broaden and build, Advances in Experimental Social Psychology, 47, 1–53.

69 people typically report fewer memory or other cognitive problems when they feel like themselves again: See S.W. Kinsinger et al. (2010), Relationship between depression, fatigue, subjective cognitive impairment, and objective neuropsychological functioning in patients with multiple sclerosis, Neuropsychology, 24, 573–580.

69 One particularly handy and evidence-based internal strategy to improve attention is verbalizing a task: For a summary of some recent research using this technique, see S.K. Kucherer and R.J. Ferguson (2017), Cognitive behavioral therapy for cancer related cognitive dysfunction, Current Opinion in Supportive and Palliative Care, 11(1), 46–51.

70 This comes from the research on ADHD: See S.A. Safren et al. (2005), Mastering Your Adult ADHD: A Cognitive-Behavioral Treatment Program, New York, NY: Oxford University Press.

71 *In particular, the flow state, as discussed by psychologist Mihaly Csiksz-entmihalyi*: See M. Csikszentmihalyi (1990), *Flow: The Psychology of Optimal Experience*, New York, NY: Harper Perennial.

74 *As Peter Brown and his colleagues write in their helpful book*: See P.C. Brown et al. (2014), *Make It Stick: The Science of Successful Learning*, Cambridge, MA: Belknap Press.

75 *Some innovative studies have looked at how drawing something compares to other memory techniques*: See J.D. Wammes et al. (2016), The drawing effect: Evidence for reliable and robust memory benefits in free recall, *Quarterly Journal of Experimental Psychology*, 69(9), 1752–1776. *Another study found a similar pattern in younger and older participants*: M.E. Meade et al. (2018), Drawing as an encoding tool: Memorial benefits in younger and older adults, *Experimental Aging Research*, 44(5), 369–396.

76 *The science indicates that these are the types of problems people report at high levels*: See A. Singh-Manoux et al. (2014), Subjective cognitive complaints and mortality: Does the type of complaint matter? *Journal of Psychiatric Research*, 48, 73–78.

80 *As we discussed earlier, research shows that multitasking*: See E. Ophir et al. (2009), Cognitive control in media multitaskers, *Proceedings of the National Academy of Sciences USA*, 106, 15583–15587.

CHAPTER 5: **What Does Exercise Do for the Brain?**

87 *Only about 20% of adults and elders exercise at levels recommended by the U.S. Department of Health and Human Services*: For recent statistics in this regard, see D.L. Blackwell and T.C. Clarke (2018), *State Variation in Meeting the 2008 Federal Guidelines for both Aerobic and Muscle-Strengthening Activities through Leisure-Time Physical Activity among Adults Aged 18–64: United States 2010–2015*, National Health Statistics Reports, no. 112, Hyattsville, MD: National Center for Health Statistics; see also Centers for Disease Control and Prevention (2013), Adult participation in aerobic and muscle-strengthening physical activities—United States, 2011, *MMWR*, 62(17), 326–330.

88 *Recent research has clarified that around the world—in 54 separate countries—excessive sitting*: See L.F. Rezende et al. (2016), All-cause mortality attributable to sitting time: Analysis of 54 countries worldwide, *American Journal of Preventative Medicine*, 51(2), 253–263.

88 *Another study found that the more hours per day you spend sitting*: See P. Siddarth et al. (2018), Sedentary behavior associated with reduced medial temporal lobe thickness in middle-aged and older adults, *PLOS ONE*, *13*(4), e0195549.

91 *the science indicates that exercise has a number of direct and indirect effects on the body's cardiovascular system*: A large recent study clarified the importance of exercise over the course of 30+ years for cardiovascular health and found particular benefits for moderate exercise; see M.F.H. Maessen et al. (2016), Lifelong exercise patterns and cardiovascular health, *Mayo Clinic Proceedings*, *91*(6), 745–754.

93 *We now know that neurons grow in response to exercise in two critically important brain regions*: As one example, see K.I. Erickson et al. (2010), Physical activity predicts gray matter volume in late adulthood, *Neurology*, *75*, 1415–1422.

93 *In one of the early studies to demonstrate how the brain responds to exercise*: As one example, see K.I. Erickson et al. (2011), Exercise training increases size of hippocampus and improves memory, *Proceedings of the National Academy of Sciences USA*, *108*(7), 3017–3022.

94 *the more their fitness improved during the study, the bigger their hippocampus got*: See L. Jonasson et al. (2017), Aerobic exercise intervention, cognitive performance, and brain structure: Results from the Physical Influences on Brain in Aging (PHIBRA) study, *Frontiers in Aging Neuroscience*, *8*, 336, doi:10.3389/fnagi.2016.00336.

95 *One area that's received a lot of attention is how neuroprotective factors such as brain-derived neurotrophic factor (BDNF)*: For a great review of this topic from a few years back, see C.W. Cotman et al. (2007), Exercise builds brain health: Key roles of growth factor cascades and inflammation, *Trends in Neurosciences*, *30*(9), 464–472.

95 *One of the interesting things about BDNF*: See K. Szuhany et al. (2015), A meta-analytic review of the effects of exercise on brain-derived neurotrophic factor, *Journal of Psychiatric Research*, *60*, 56–64.

95 *Some research has even highlighted a connection between inflammation and Alzheimer's disease*: See M.T. Heneka et al. (2015), Neuroinflammation in Alzheimer's disease, *Lancet Neurology*, *14*(4), 388–405; see also Q. Tao et al. (2018), Association of chronic low-grade inflammation with risk of Alzheimer disease in ApoE4 carriers, *JAMA Network Open*, *1*(6), e183597.

96 *there's evidence that higher physical fitness and exercise levels reduce*

inflammation: See J. Hwang et al. (2017), The positive cognitive impact of aerobic fitness is associated with peripheral inflammatory and brain-derived neurotrophic biomarkers in young adults, *Physiology & Behavior, 179*, 75–89; see also F. Lin et al. (2012), Effect of leisure activities on inflammation and cognitive function in an aging sample, *Archives of Gerontology and Geriatrics, 54*, e398–e404; and C.W. Cotman et al. (2007) as noted above.

96 *physical inactivity is a "modifiable risk factor" that is associated with more cases of Alzheimer's disease*: See D.E. Barnes and K. Yaffe (2011), The projected impact of risk factor reduction on Alzheimer's disease prevalence, *Lancet Neurology, 10*(9), 819–828.

96 *the risk gets progressively lower the more types of physical activity you engage in*: A very creative and interesting study found that 4+ types of physical activity (including things like walking, gardening, hiking, biking, or dancing) was better than just one type in preventing dementia over a 5-year period; see L.J. Podewils et al. (2005), Physical activity, APOE genotype, and dementia risk: Findings from the Cardiovascular Health Cognition Study, *American Journal of Epidemiology, 161*(7), 639–651.

97 *The findings indicated that for every 1,000 steps walked*: See V. Varma et al. (2015), Low-intensity daily walking activity is associated with hippocampal volume in older adults, *Hippocampus, 25*, 605–615.

97 *Other research has found that walking 6 to 9 miles per week*: See K.I. Erickson et al. (2010) above.

98 *yoga can promote richer connections throughout the brain and improve memory*: See H.A. Eyre et al (2016), Changes in neural connectivity and memory following a yoga intervention for older adults: A pilot study, *Journal of Alzheimer's Disease, 52*, 673–684; regarding tai chi, see G. Zheng (2015), Tai Chi and the protection of cognitive ability: A systematic review of prospective studies in healthy adults, *American Journal of Preventative Medicine, 49*(1), 89–97.

98 *There's also evidence that aqua aerobics . . . and cycling*: See C.T. Albinet et al. (2016), Executive function improvement following a 5-month aquaerobics program in older adults: Role of cardiac vagal control in inhibition performance, *Biological Psychology, 115*, 69–77; see also M. Roig et al. (2016), Time-dependent effects of cardiovascular exercise on memory, *Exercise and Sport Sciences Reviews, 44*(2), 81–88.

98 *moderately intense activity is the sweet spot for heart-related benefits*: See M.F.H. Maessen et al. (2016), above.

98 *one study found that walking or jogging 75 minutes per week ramped up attention and visual–spatial skills:* See E.D. Vidoni et al. (2015), Dose-response of aerobic exercise on cognition: A community-based, pilot randomized controlled trial, *PLOS ONE, 10*(7), e0131647.

99 *Other research has found that from our teens to our seventies, exercising up to 2 hours per week benefits executive functioning:* See B. Gaertner et al. (2018), Physical exercise and cognitive function across the lifespan: Results of a nationwide population-based study, *Journal of Science and Medicine in Sport, 21*, 489–494.

99 *A massive recent study—involving over 100,000 people across 20 countries:* See P. de Souto Barreto et al. (2016), Physical activity and cognitive function in middle-aged and older adults: An analysis of 104,909 people from 20 countries, *Mayo Clinic Proceedings, 91*, 1515–1524.

100 *individual exercise sessions have been found to temporarily improve our focus and executive functioning skills:* For a recent study examining acute effects of physical activity on cognition, see A. Dunsky et al. (2017), The effects of a resistance vs. an aerobic single session on attention and executive functioning in adults, *PLOS ONE, 12*(4), e0176092; see also J.C. Basso et al. (2015), Acute exercise improves prefrontal cortex but not hippocampal function in healthy adults, *Journal of the International Neuropsychological Society, 21*, 791–801.

100 *A reasonable answer comes from a study that reviewed about 100 clinical trials:* See J. Gomes-Osman et al. (2018), Exercise for cognitive brain health in aging: A systematic review for an evaluation of dose, *Neurology: Clinical Practice, 8*(3), 1–9.

101 *people tend to process information more efficiently and be less error-prone after a period of HIIT:* See C.R.R. Alves et al. (2014), Influence of acute high-intensity aerobic interval exercise bout on selective attention and short-term memory tasks, *Perceptual and Motor Skills, 118*(1), 63–72; see also S.-C. Kao et al. (2017), Comparison of the acute effects of high-intensity interval training and continuous aerobic walking on inhibitory control, *Psychophysiology, 54*, 1335–1345.

101 *HIIT may also boost executive functioning skills for a longer period than moderate exercise:* See H. Tsukamoto et al. (2016), Greater impact of acute high-intensity interval exercise on post-exercise executive function compared to moderate-intensity continuous exercise, *Physiology & Behavior, 155*, 224–230; see also J. Hwang et al. (2016),

Acute high-intensity exercise-induced cognitive enhancement and brain-derived neurotrophic factor in young, healthy adults, *Neuroscience Letters, 630,* 247–253.

101 *HIIT has also been found to enhance physical fitness:* See K. Weston et al. (2014), High-intensity interval training in patients with lifestyle-induced cardiometabolic disease: A systematic review and meta-analysis, *British Journal of Sports Medicine, 48,* 1227–1234.

101 *We know that beginning to exercise at any point in life:* See Q. Tian et al. (2014), Physical activity predicts microstructural integrity in memory-related networks in very old adults, *Journals of Gerontology, Series A: Biological Sciences and Medical Sciences, 69*(10), 1284–1290; see also S.J. Colcombe et al. (2006), Aerobic exercise training increases brain volume in aging humans, *Journals of Gerontology, Series A: Biological Sciences and Medical Sciences, 61*(11), 1166–1170.

102 *Multiple studies have shown that the more fit we are in midlife:* See J. Kulmala et al. (2014), Association between mid- to late life physical fitness and dementia: Evidence from the CAIDE study, *Journal of Internal Medicine, 276,* 296–307; see also S. Rovio et al. (2005), Leisure-time physical activity at midlife and the risk of dementia and Alzheimer's disease, *Lancet Neurology, 4,* 705–711; N.L. Spartano et al. (2016), Midlife exercise blood pressure, heart rate, and fitness related to brain volume 2 decades later, *Neurology, 86,* 1–7.

102 *any level of physical activity is associated with a lower risk of cognitive impairment:* See F. Sofi et al. (2011), Physical activity and risk of cognitive decline: A meta-analysis of prospective studies, *Journal of Internal Medicine, 269,* 107–117.

102 *Even in the near term, stronger cardiovascular fitness in middle age is associated with more brain volume:* See N. Zhu et al. (2015), Cardiorespiratory fitness and brain volume and white matter integrity, *Neurology, 84,* 1–7.

102 *One of the longest studies examining exercise and the brain:* See H. Horder et al. (2018), Midlife cardiovascular fitness and dementia, *Neurology, 90*(15), e1298–e1305, doi:10.1212/WNL.0000000000005290.

103 *recent research followed a group of over 3,000 children and adolescents:* See S. Rovio et al. (2017), Cardiovascular risk factors from childhood and midlife cognitive performance: The Young Finns Study, *Journal of the American College of Cardiology, 69,* 2279–2289.

103 *The executive functions of the brain . . . also really respond to exercise:* See E. Cox et al. (2016), Relationship between physical activity

and cognitive function in apparently healthy young to middle-aged adults: A systematic review, *Journal of Science and Medicine in Sport*, *19*, 616–628.

103 *this biological profile of sorts is also associated with reduced executive functioning*: See S. Kaur et al. (2016), Serum brain-derived neurotrophic factor mediates the relationship between abdominal adiposity and executive function in middle age, *Journal of the International Neuropsychological Society*, *22*, 1–8.

104 *People who maintain a consistent exercise habit are often internally motivated to do so, but also tend to have a friend who is pretty active*: See E. Burton et al. (2018), Effectiveness of peers in delivering programs or motivating older people to increase their participation in physical activity: Systematic review and meta-analysis, *Journal of Sports Sciences*, *36*(6), 666–678; see also I. Janssen et al. (2014), Correlates of 15-year maintenance of physical activity in middle-aged women, *International Journal of Behavioral Medicine*, *21*, 511–518.

104 *what you look at while exercising really seems to matter*: See M. Rogerson et al. (2016), Influences of green outdoors versus indoors environmental settings on psychological and social outcomes of controlled exercise, *International Journal of Environmental Research and Public Health*, *13*(4), 363, doi:10.3390/ijerph13040363; see also J. Kowal and M.S. Fortier (2007), Physical activity behavior change in middle-aged and older women: The role of barriers and of environmental characteristics, *Journal of Behavioral Medicine*, *30*, 233–242.

105 *When physical activity is prioritized definitively in this way*: See W. Miller and P.R. Brown (2017), Motivators, facilitators, and barriers to physical activity in older adults, *Holistic Nurse Practitioner*, *31*, 216–224.

CHAPTER 6: **Socializing and the Brain: Stay Connected to Improve Your Neural Connections**

112 *It also improves our overall health and affects our basic physiology across the life span*: See Y.C. Yang et al. (2016), Social relationships and physiological determinants of longevity across the human life span, *Proceedings of the National Academy of Sciences USA*, *113*(3), 578–583.

113 *people who feel more supported have lower blood pressure*: See B.N. Uchino et al. (1996), The relationship between social support and

physiological processes: A review with emphasis on underlying mechanisms and implications for health, *Psychological Bulletin*, *119*, 488–531; see also Y.C. Yang et al. (2016) above.

113 *The size of our social network is also linked to health*: See S. Cohen and D. Janicki-Devert (2009), Can we improve our physical health by altering our social networks? *Perspectives on Psychological Science*, *4*, 375–378.

113 *negative encounters tend to stir up brain regions that are active when we experience physical pain*: See N.I. Eisenberger (2012), The pain of social disconnection: Examining the shared neural underpinnings of physical and social pain, *Nature Reviews Neuroscience*, *13*, 421–434.

115 *emotional support from others quiets the parts of the brain that light up when we feel threatened*: For a great review of this area of research, see N.I. Eisenberger (2013), An empirical review of the neural underpinnings of receiving and giving social support: Implications for health, *Psychosomatic Medicine*, *75*, 545–556.

115 *after considering effects of physical and mental activity, people who were most socially active*: See B.D. James et al. (2011), Late-life social activity and cognitive decline in old age, *Journal of the International Neuropsychological Society*, *17*, 998–1005.

116 *Other research has found that social activity can enhance our executive function skills*: See C.M. deFrias and R.A. Dixon (2014), Lifestyle engagement affects cognitive status differences and trajectories on executive functions in older adults, *Archives of Clinical Neuropsychology*, *29*, 16–25.

116 *there's also evidence that being more social makes us feel like our memory is better*: See H. Litwin and K.J. Stoeckel (2016), Social network, activity participation, and cognition: A complex relationship, *Research on Aging*, *38*(1), 76–97.

116 *people who have more socially active jobs are less likely to develop cognitive problems such as dementia*: See E.A. Boots et al. (2015), Occupational complexity and cognitive reserve in a middle-aged cohort at risk for Alzheimer's disease, *Archives of Clinical Neuropsychology*, *30*(7), 634–642.

116 *there's evidence that we can make up for being less social at work*: See R. Andel et al. (2014), The role of midlife occupational complexity and leisure activity in late life cognition, *Journals of Gerontology, Series B: Psychological Sciences and Social Sciences*, *70*, 314–321.

117 *scientists gauged how often people were in touch with friends or family members*: See A.R. Teo et al. (2015), Does mode of contact with different types of social relationships predict depression in older adults? Evidence from a nationally representative survey, *Journal of the American Geriatrics Society, 63*, 2014–2022.

118 *Some of the early knowledge in this area came from the so-called Nun Study*: For a detailed description of this study and its findings, see D. Snowdon (2001), *Aging with Grace: What the Nun Study Teaches Us About Leading Longer, Healthier, and More Meaningful Lives*, New York, NY: Bantam Books.

119 *Some of the more compelling studies have found that the more people you connect with on a regular or semi-regular basis*: As one early example, see R.E. Holtzman et al. (2004), Social network characteristics and cognition in middle-aged and older adults, *Journals of Gerontology, Series B: Psychological Sciences and Social Sciences, 59B*(6), P278–P284.

119 *the less likely you'll show cognitive decline, and the longer you'll live*: See J. Holt-Lunstad et al. (2010), Social relationships and mortality risk: A meta-analytic review, *PLOS Medicine, 7*(7), e1000316, doi:10.1371/journal.pmed.1000316.

119 *A study from the Rush Alzheimer's Disease Center sought to understand whether a larger social network*: See L.L. Barnes et al. (2004), Social resources and cognitive decline in a population of older African Americans and whites, *Neurology, 63*, 2322–2326.

119 *Other work has shown that the risk of dementia is quite high in those with few or no consistent social contacts*: See L. Fratiglioni et al. (2000), Influence of social network on occurrence of dementia: A community-based longitudinal study, *Lancet, 355*, 1315–1319.

119 *A fascinating study tried to determine whether social networks could buffer the effects of pathological changes*: See D.A. Bennett et al. (2006), The effect of social networks on the relation between Alzheimer's disease pathology and level of cognitive function in old people: A longitudinal cohort study, *Lancet Neurology, 5*(5), 406–412.

120 *Some research has found that the more satisfied we are with others in our social networks*: See H. Amieva et al. (2010), What aspects of social network are protective for dementia? Not the quantity but the quality of social interactions is protective up to 15 years later, *Psychosomatic Medicine, 72*, 905–911.

122 *An early study in this area looked at the effects of social support on*

cognitive aging: See T.E. Seeman et al. (2001), Social relationships, social support, and patterns of cognitive aging in healthy, high-functioning older adults: MacArthur studies of successful aging, *Health Psychology*, 20, 243–255.

122 *While some work has found that more social support is related to better overall cognitive functioning*: A variety of studies have clarified these relationships. See K.R. Krueger et al. (2009), Social engagement and cognitive function in old age, *Experimental Aging Research*, 35, 45–60; see also T.E. Seeman et al. (2011), Histories of social engagement and adult cognition: Midlife in the U.S. study, *Journals of Gerontology, Series B: Psychological Sciences and Social Sciences*, 66B, i141–i152; L.B. Zahodne et al. (2014), Which psychosocial factors best predict cognitive performance in older adults? *Journal of the International Neuropsychological Society*, 20, 487–495; and M.L. Zuelsdorff et al. (2013), Stressful events, social support, and cognitive function in middle-aged adults with a family history of Alzheimer's disease, *Journal of Aging Health*, 25, 944–959.

123 *Some research has found that our sense of being supported well by others*: See T.F. Hughes (2008), The association between social resources and cognitive change in older adults: Evidence from the Charlotte County Healthy Aging Study, *Journal of Gerontology: Psychological Sciences*, 63B(4), P241–P244.

123 *feeling the scales of social reciprocity tipping in our favor*: See H. Amieva et al. (2010) above.

123 *A large study that followed over 3,000 Mexican Americans over about 7 years*: See T.D. Hill et al. (2006), Religious attendance and cognitive functioning among older Mexican Americans, *Journals of Gerontology, Series B: Psychological Sciences and Social Sciences*, 61(1), P3–P9.

124 *volunteering helps the brain work better*: See S. Park et al. (2017), Life course trajectories of later-life cognitive functions: Does social engagement in old age matter? *International Journal of Environmental Research and Public Health*, 14(4), 393, doi:10.3390/ijerph14040393.

124 *a study that examined whether participating in a volunteer program for elementary school children*: See M.C. Carlson et al. (2008), Exploring the effects of an "everyday" activity program on executive function and memory in older adults: Experience Corps, *Gerontologist*, 48(6), 793–801; see also M.C. Carlson et al. (2009), Evidence for neurocognitive plasticity in at-risk older adults: The Experience Corps program, *Journals of Gerontology, Series A: Biological Sciences*

and Medical Sciences, 64, 1275–1282; M.C. Carlson et al. (2015), Impact of the Baltimore Experience Corps Trial on cortical and hippocampal volumes, *Alzheimer's & Dementia*, 11, 1340–1348.

126 *we know that individuals who consistently have negative interactions are less able to regulate cortisol*: See K.S. Rook (2015), Social networks in later life: Weighing positive and negative effects on health and well-being, *Current Directions in Psychological Science*, 24(1), 45–51.

126 *One study followed middle-aged people over a 10-year period*: See J. Liao et al. (2014), Negative aspects of close relationships as risk factors for cognitive aging, *American Journal of Epidemiology*, 180, 1118–1125.

127 *research finds negative effects of social isolation on the immune system*: See Y.C. Yang et al. (2016) above.

127 *the health-oriented effects of isolation are not unlike those related to obesity or smoking*: See A. Richard et al. (2017), Loneliness is adversely associated with physical and mental health and lifestyle factors: Results from a Swiss national survey, *PLOS ONE*, 12(7), e0181442.

127 *older adults who are socially isolated are significantly more likely to die prematurely*: See P.M. Eng et al. (2002), Social ties and change in social ties in relation to subsequent total and cause-specific mortality and coronary heart disease incidence in men, *American Journal of Epidemiology*, 155(8), 700–709.

127 *people who report loneliness have been found to show more rapid cognitive decline than others*: See N.J. Donovan et al. (2017), Loneliness, depression and cognitive function in older U.S. adults, *International Journal of Geriatric Psychiatry*, 32(5), 564–573; see also R.S. Wilson et al. (2007), Loneliness and risk of Alzheimer disease, *Archives of General Psychiatry*, 64, 234–240.

127 *those with a limited social network show a significantly increased risk of developing cognitive impairment*: See L. Fratiglioni et al. (2000) above; see also S.S. Bassuk et al. (1999), Social disengagement and incident cognitive decline in community-dwelling elderly persons, *Annals of Internal Medicine*, 31(3), 165–173.

CHAPTER 7: The Benefits of Giving Your Brain a Workout: Mental Activities and Hobbies to Embrace

134 *we see that people without a lot of early-life education*: See M.E. Lachman et al. (2010), Frequent cognitive activity compensates for

education differences in episodic memory, *American Journal of Geriatric Psychiatry, 18*(1), 4–10.

135 *A promising early study followed more than 1,700 cognitively healthy people over time*: See N. Scarmeas et al. (2001), Influence of leisure activity on the incidence of Alzheimer's disease, *Neurology, 57,* 2236–2242.

135 *Other seminal research—an extension of the classic Nun Study*: R.S. Wilson et al. (2002), Participation in cognitively stimulating activities and risk of incident Alzheimer disease, *JAMA, 287*(6), 742–748.

136 *And a review and meta-analysis of many studies in this area*: See L.A. Yates et al. (2016), Cognitive leisure activities and future risk of cognitive impairment and dementia: Systematic review and meta-analysis, *International Psychogeriatrics, 28*(11), 1791–1806.

136 *being involved with a hobby of interest is associated with better overall health*: See S.D. Pressman et al. (2009), Association of enjoyable leisure activities with psychological and physical well-being, *Psychosomatic Medicine, 71*(7), 725–732.

136 *less mental activity has been linked to atrophy of the medial temporal lobe*: See D. Yoshida et al. (2012), The relationship between atrophy of the medial temporal area and daily activities in older adults with mild cognitive impairment, *Aging Clinical and Experimental Research, 24*(5), 423–429.

136 *reading books, newspapers, or magazines has been found to be particularly important in reducing dementia risk*: See N. Scarmeas et al. (2001) above.

136 *Reading on a regular basis might even have a more protective effect on the brain than the years of education*: See M.A. Lopes et al. (2012), High prevalence of dementia in a community-based survey of older people from Brazil: Association with intellectual activity rather than education, *Journal of Alzheimer's Disease, 32*(2), 307–316; see also M.E. Lachman et al. (2010) above.

137 *Other studies have found that reading reduces the risk of developing milder cognitive problems*: See Y.E. Geda et al. (2011), Engaging in cognitive activities, aging and mild cognitive impairment: A population-based study, *Journal of Neuropsychiatry and Clinical Neurosciences, 23*(2), 149–154.

137 *and improves our ability to appreciate others' perspectives*: For a study examining the role of reading fiction and nonfiction on *theory of*

mind (our ability to take others' perspectives in different ways), see D.C. Kidd and E. Castano (2013), Reading literary fiction improves theory of mind, *Science, 342*(6156), 377–380.

137 *a specific study that supports the powerful brain effects of being a cruciverbalist*: See J.A. Pillai et al. (2011), Association of crossword puzzle participation with memory decline in persons who develop dementia, *Journal of the International Neuropsychological Society, 17*, 1006–1013; see also T. Hughes et al. (2010), Engagement in reading and hobbies and risk of incident dementia: The MoVIES Project, *American Journal of Alzheimer's Disease and Other Dementias, 25*(5), 432–438.

138 *Maybe you like playing cards or checkers*: See E. Jonaitis et al. (2013), Cognitive activities and cognitive performance in middle-aged adults at risk for Alzheimer's disease, *Psychology and Aging, 28*(4), 1004–1014.

138 *Another study investigated common leisure activities like reading*: J. Verghese et al. (2003), Leisure activities and the risk of dementia in the elderly, *New England Journal of Medicine, 348*(25), 2508–2516.

139 *A study from scientists at the University of Southern California looked at pairs of twins*: See M.A. Balbag et al. (2014), Playing a musical instrument as a protective factor against dementia and cognitive impairment: A population-based twin study, *International Journal of Alzheimer's Disease, 2014*(8 suppl 4), article ID 836748, doi:10.1155/2014/836748.

140 *Other studies have found that the more musically engaged one is throughout life*: See B. Hanna-Pladdy and A. McKay (2011), The relation between instrumental musical activity and cognitive aging, *Neuropsychology, 25*(3), 378–386; see also J.A. Bugos (2007), Individualized piano instruction enhances executive functioning and working memory in older adults, *Aging & Mental Health, 11*(4), 464–471.

140 *One study trained people in digital photography techniques, quilting, or both*: See D.C. Park et al. (2014), The impact of sustained engagement on cognitive function in older adults: The Synapse Project, *Psychological Science, 25*(1), 103–112; see also Y.E. Geda et al. (2011) above.

141 *the wider the variety of activities, the more benefits these women reaped*: See M.C. Carlson et al. (2012), Lifestyle activities and memory: Variety may be the spice of life. The Women's Health and Aging

Study II, *Journal of the International Neuropsychological Society*, 18, 286–294.

141 *these researchers found something similar for exercise*: See L.J. Podewils et al. (2005), Physical activity, APOE genotype, and dementia risk: Findings from the Cardiovascular Health Cognition Study, *American Journal of Epidemiology*, 161(7), 639–651.

142 *One study found that over time, people who regularly sought out novel and mentally stimulating activities*: See T. Fritsch et al. (2005), Participation in novelty-seeking leisure activities and Alzheimer's disease, *Journal of Geriatric Psychiatry & Neurology*, 18, 134–141.

142 *reducing the time one spends on intellectual hobbies from young adulthood to middle age increases the risk of Alzheimer's disease*: See R.P. Friedland et al. (2001), Patients with Alzheimer's disease have reduced activities in midlife compared with healthy control-group members, *Proceedings of the National Academy of Sciences USA*, 98(6), 3440–3445.

142 *while participating in one type of activity was helpful, an increased "dose" of two or more activities*: See A. Karp et al. (2006), Mental, physical and social components in leisure activities equally contribute to decrease dementia risk, *Dementia and Geriatric Cognitive Disorders*, 21, 65–73.

142 *there seems to be evidence that spending at least an hour per day is particularly effective*: See T. Hughes et al. (2010) above.

143 *If you're in your forties, another study might motivate you to keep your brain firing*: See M.C. Carlson et al. (2008), Midlife activity predicts risk of dementia in older male twin pairs, *Alzheimer's & Dementia*, 4, 324–331.

144 *A large study followed people for about 20 years who began the research in in their late fifties*: See I. Kareholt et al. (2011), Baseline leisure activity and cognition more than two decades later, *International Journal of Geriatric Psychiatry*, 26, 65–74.

144 *A study from a few years ago looked at the complexity of one's job in three domains*: See E. Boots et al. (2015), Occupational complexity and cognitive reserve in a middle-aged cohort at risk for Alzheimer's disease, *Archives of Clinical Neuropsychology*, 30, 634–642.

145 *Some research has found that people can in a sense make up for a cognitively dull job*: See R. Andel et al. (2014), The role of midlife occupational complexity and leisure activity in late-life cognition, *Journals*

of Gerontology, Series B: Psychological Sciences and Social Sciences, 70(2), 314–321.

146 *In a comprehensive review of the science to date:* See D.J. Simons et al. (2016), Do "brain-training" programs work? *Psychological Science in the Public Interest, 17*(3), 103–186.

146 *A recent meta-analysis that examined more than 300 studies in this area:* See G. Sala et al. (2018), Video game training does not enhance cognitive ability: A comprehensive meta-analytic investigation, *Psychological Bulletin, 144*(2), 111–139.

147 *One study recruited people by using two types of flyers:* See C.K. Foroughi et al. (2016), Placebo effects in cognitive training, *Proceedings of the National Academy of Sciences USA, 113*(27), 7470–7474, doi:10.1073/pnas.1601243113.

147 *And some scientists do see the potential for brain games to augment our cognitive skills:* More than 130 scientists wrote a letter in response to an earlier scientist consensus criticizing brain training games. See Cognitive Training Data (2015), Open letter response to the Stanford Center on Longevity, available at https://www .cognitivetrainingdata.org/the-controversy-does-brain-training -work/response-letter/. Compare this position to the earlier letter, signed by over 70 scientists: Stanford Center on Longevity (2014), A consensus on the brain training industry from the scientific community, available at http://longevity3.stanford.edu/ blog/2014/10/15/the-consensus-on-the-brain-training-industry -from-the-scientific-community-2/.

CHAPTER 8: Your Brain Is What You Eat: Nutrition and Cognition

156 *recent research has found that losing weight doesn't necessarily impact overall mortality:* See V.W. Barry et al. (2014), Fitness vs. fatness on all-cause mortality: A meta-analysis, *Progress in Cardiovascular Diseases, 56*, 382–390.

157 *In 2017, AARP conducted a study that clarified dietary habits:* See L. Mehegan et al. (2018), *2017 Brain Health and Nutrition Survey,* Washington DC: AARP Research, https://doi.org/10.26419/res .00187.001.

158 *Some of the common barriers include high cost:* In addition to the AARP study mentioned above, one study specifically looked at barriers to eating fruits and vegetables, and what facilitates such consumption: M.-C. Yeh et al. (2008), Understanding barriers and facilitators of fruit and vegetable consumption among a diverse

multi-ethnic population in the USA, *Health Promotion International*, *23*(1), 42–51.

159   *The diet is mostly plant-based and consists of lots of fruits and vegetables*: For an updated scientific consensus on what constitutes the main components of the Mediterranean diet, see A. Bach-Faig et al. (2011), Mediterranean diet pyramid today. Science and cultural updates, *Public Health Nutrition, 14*(12A), 2274–2284.

159   *A wide variety of nutritional studies reveal the same thing*: See I. Lourida et al. (2013), Mediterranean diet, cognitive function, and dementia: A systematic review, *Epidemiology, 24*, 479–489; B. Singh et al. (2014), Association of Mediterranean diet with mild cognitive impairment and Alzheimer's disease: A systematic review and meta-analysis, *Journal of Alzheimer's Disease, 39*(2), 271–282; and V. Solfrizzi et al. (2017), Relationships of dietary patterns, foods, and micro- and macronutrients with Alzheimer's disease and late-life cognitive disorders: A systematic review, *Journal of Alzheimer's Disease, 59*, 815–849.

160   *There is also less risk of converting from MCI to dementia*: See B. Singh et al. (2014) above.

160   *there's a lower risk of stroke and depression in those who follow a Mediterranean-style diet*: See T. Psaltopoulou et al. (2013), Mediterranean diet, stroke, cognitive impairment, and depression: A meta-analysis, *Annals of Neurology, 74*, 580–591.

160   *One study a few years ago evaluated the diets of over 2,000 people*: See N. Scarmeas et al. (2006), Mediterranean diet and risk of Alzheimer's disease, *Annals of Neurology, 59*(6), 912–921.

161   *A large group of older adults was asked how much they exercised and how much they adhered to the MeDi*: See N. Scarmeas et al. (2009), Physical activity, diet, and risk of Alzheimer disease, *JAMA, 302*(6), 627–637.

162   *The diet may also have antithrombotic and antiatherogenic features*: See T. Psaltopoulou et al. (2013) above.

162   *People adhering to the MeDi have denser brain matter in multiple regions*: Multiple recent studies have clarified the brain-related benefits of the MeDi. See S.C. Staubo et al. (2017), Mediterranean diet, micronutrients and macronutrients, and MRI measures of cortical thickness, *Alzheimer's & Dementia, 13*, 168–177; M. Luciano et al. (2017), Mediterranean-type diet and brain structural change from 73 to 76 years in a Scottish cohort, *Neurology, 88*, 449–455; and L. Mosconi et al. (2018), Lifestyle and vascular risk effects on MRI-based biomark-

ers of Alzheimer's disease: A cross-sectional study of middle-aged adults from the broader New York City area, *BMJ Open*, 8, e019362.

162 *Less dietary intake of red meat and dairy products, and more fish consumption*: See Y. Gu et al. (2015), Mediterranean diet and brain structure in a multiethnic elderly cohort, *Neurology*, 85, 1744–1751.

163 *People eating the MeDi also have brain regions showing better structural connectivity*: See A. Pelletier et al. (2015), Mediterranean diet and preserved brain structural connectivity in older subjects, *Alzheimer's & Dementia*, 11, 1023–1031.

163 *people eating in a DASH style have been found to show better overall cognitive functioning and quicker thinking speed*: See P.J. Smith et al. (2010), Effects of the Dietary Approaches to Stop Hypertension diet and caloric restriction on neurocognition in overweight adults with high blood pressure, *Hypertension*, 55, 1331–1338; see also H. Wengreen et al. (2013), Prospective study of Dietary Approaches to Stop Hypertension- and Mediterranean-style dietary patterns and age-related cognitive change: The Cache County Study on Memory, Health and Aging, *American Journal of Clinical Nutrition*, 98, 1263–1271.

163 *They also have a reduced risk of developing Alzheimer's disease*: See M.C. Morris et al. (2015a), MIND diet associated with reduced incidence of Alzheimer's disease, *Alzheimer's & Dementia*, 11, 1007–1014.

163 *Another study created what was termed a healthy eating index*: See A. Smyth et al. (2015), Healthy eating and reduced risk of cognitive decline, *Neurology*, 84, 2258–2265.

164 *An additional dietary style that is associated with cognitive health is what researchers have called a prudent diet*: See B. Shakersain et al. (2016), Prudent diet may attenuate the adverse effects of Western diet on cognitive decline, *Alzheimer's & Dementia*, 12, 100–109.

165 *To be fair, many people enjoy hamburgers and fish*: The AARP study described earlier actually found that this is a very common dietary tendency: 37% of people in their survey reported eating both fish and red meat in a typical week, which was more common than just eating red meat (29%) or just eating seafood (15%).

165 *Some research suggests that this dietary style, which is high in saturated fat and refined sugar*: See H. Francis and R. Stevenson (2013), The longer-term impacts of Western diet on human cognition and the brain, *Appetite*, 63, 119–128; see also A. Knight et al. (2016), Is

the Mediterranean diet a feasible approach to preserving cognitive function and reducing risk of dementia for older adults in Western countries? New insights and future directions, *Ageing Research Reviews*, 25, 85–101.

166 *One study from a few years ago assessed fruit and vegetable consumption in a large sample of older women*: J.H. Kang et al. (2005), Fruit and vegetable consumption and cognitive decline in aging women, *Annals of Neurology*, 57, 713–720.

167 *Another study found something similar: consuming leafy vegetables was linked to slower cognitive decline*: See M.C. Morris et al. (2006), Associations of vegetable and fruit consumption with age-related cognitive change, *Neurology*, 67, 1370–1376.

167 *Some recent nutritional research has further clarified the connection between vegetables and cognition*: See M.C. Morris et al. (2018), Nutrients and bioactives in green leafy vegetables and cognitive decline, *Neurology*, 90, e214–e222.

168 *Only about 10% of people have a serving of vegetables each day*: See S.H. Lee-Kwan et al. (2017), Disparities in state-specific adult fruit and vegetable consumption—United States, 2015, *Morbidity and Mortality Weekly Report*, 66(45), 1241–1247.

168 *Flavonoids are thought to be particularly important for the brain given their antioxidant properties*: See E.E. Devore et al. (2012), Dietary intake of berries and flavonoids in relation to cognitive decline, *Annals of Neurology*, 72(1), 135–143.

168 *Human research has shown that people who eat more berries show less cognitive decline, better working memory, and increased blood flow in multiple brain regions*: See J.L. Bowtell et al. (2017), Enhanced task-related brain activation and resting perfusion in healthy older adults after chronic blueberry supplementation, *Applied Physiology, Nutrition, and Metabolism*, 42, 773–779.

168 *They also tend to report fewer problems with executive functioning skills in daily life*: See R.K. McNamara et al. (2018), Cognitive response to fish oil, blueberry, and combined supplementation in older adults with subjective cognitive impairment, *Neurobiology of Aging*, 64, 147–156.

168 *The largest study to date looking at blueberries and cognition enrolled more than 16,000 older women*: See E.E. Devore et al. (2012) above.

169 *a relatively new dietary style builds on the Mediterranean diet and emphasizes berry and green leafy vegetable intake*: See A.M. Berend-

sen et al. (2018), Association of long-term adherence to the MIND diet with cognitive function and cognitive decline in American women, *Journal of Nutrition, Health and Aging, 22*(2), 222–229; see also M.C. Morris et al. (2015a) above.

169 *It can also slow the process of cognitive aging*: M.C. Morris et al. (2015b), MIND diet slows cognitive decline with aging, *Alzheimer's & Dementia, 11*, 1015–1022.

169 *researchers asked a group of older adults how much fish they ate*: See C.A. Raji et al. (2014), Regular fish consumption and age-related brain gray matter loss, *American Journal of Preventive Medicine, 47*(4), 444–451.

170 *Other studies indicate that the more baked or broiled fish you eat*: A few older studies looked at fish consumption and the brain. See J.K. Virtanen et al. (2008), Fish consumption and risk of subclinical brain abnormalities on MRI in older adults, *Neurology, 71*, 439–446; see also D. Mozaffarian et al. (2005), Fish consumption and stroke risk in elderly individuals: The Cardiovascular Health Study, *Archives of Internal Medicine, 165*(2), 200–206.

171 *PUFAs do many things to promote brain health*: See C. Phillips (2017), Lifestyle modulators of neuroplasticity: How physical activity, mental engagement, and diet promote cognitive health during aging, *Neural Plasticity*, article ID 3589271, doi:10.1155/2017/3589271.

171 *PUFA levels in the body are associated with more brain volume in multiple regions*: For a particularly large and impressive study in this area, see J.V. Pottala et al. (2014), Higher RBC EPA + DHA corresponds with larger total brain and hippocampal volumes, *Neurology, 82*, 435–442; see also S.M. Conklin et al. (2007), Long-chain omega-3 fatty acid intake is associated positively with corticolimbic gray matter volume in healthy adults, *Neuroscience Letters, 421*, 209–212.

171 *One study found that higher levels of one of the marine PUFAs, DHA, was associated with a 47% lower risk of any type of dementia*: See E.J. Schaefer et al. (2006), Plasma phosphatidylcholine docosahexaenoic acid content and risk of dementia and Alzheimer disease, *Archives of Neurology, 63*, 1545–1550.

172 *Beyond concerns about dementia, midlife DHA levels are correlated with better mental flexibility*: M.F. Muldoon et al. (2010), Serum phospholipid docosahexaenoic acid is associated with cognitive functioning during middle adulthood, *Journal of Nutrition, 140*, 848–853.

172 *Comprehensive reviews and meta-analyses of existing PUFA studies have mostly concluded that PUFA supplementation*: See E. Sydenham et al. (2012), Omega 3 fatty acid for the prevention of cognitive decline and dementia, *Cochrane Database of Systematic Reviews*, 6, CD005379; see also J. Jiao et al. (2014), Effect of n-3 PUFA supplementation on cognitive function throughout the life span from infancy to old age: A systematic review and meta-analysis of randomized controlled trials, *American Journal of Clinical Nutrition*, 100, 1422–1436.

172 *a recent yearlong randomized clinical trial comparing PUFAs and placebo pills in older adults*: J. Baleztena et al. (2018), Association between cognitive function and supplementation with omega-3 PUFAs and other nutrients in ≥ 75 years old patients: A randomized multicenter study, *PLOS ONE*, *13*(3), e0193568.

172 *PUFAs also do not seem to help individuals who have been diagnosed with dementia*: See M. Burckhardt et al. (2016), Omega-3 fatty acids for the treatment of dementia, *Cochrane Database of Systematic Reviews*, 4, CD009002.

172 *While a few studies have found mild cognitive benefits from taking PUFA supplements*: As one example where benefits were seen in adults with memory complaints (but not in adults without complaints), see K. Yurko-Mauro et al. (2015), Docosahexaenoic acid and adult memory: A systematic review and meta-analysis, *PLOS ONE*, *10*(3), e0120391.

173 *This is also the case regarding cardiovascular health*: See T. Aung et al. (2018), Associations of omega-3 fatty acid supplement use with cardiovascular disease risks, *JAMA Cardiology*, *3*(3), 225–234.

173 *Large individual studies and reviews of smaller studies have generally not found a consistent benefit*: Some studies in this area include E.E. Devore et al. (2013), The association of antioxidants and cognition in the nurses' health study, *American Journal of Epidemiology*, *177*(1), 33–41; and G.E. Crichton et al. (2013), Dietary antioxidants, cognitive function and dementia—A systematic review, *Plant Foods and Human Nutrition*, 68, 279–292.

173 *There have been some encouraging findings linking curcumin to improved neurological health*: See C. Phillips (2017) above.

174 *A recent study that reviewed about 40 individual studies of compounds such as ginkgo biloba*: See M. Butler et al. (2018), Over-the-counter supplement interventions to prevent cognitive decline, mild cog-

nitive impairment, and clinical Alzheimer-type dementia: A systematic review, *Annals of Internal Medicine*, 168, 52–62.

174 *A meta-analysis examining the effects of ginkgo biloba on dementia did find some benefits compared to placebo*: See M. Hashiguchi et al. (2015), Meta-analysis of the efficacy and safety of Ginkgo biloba extract for the treatment of dementia, *Journal of Pharmaceutical Health Care and Sciences*, 1(14), doi:10.1186/s40780-015-0014-7.

CHAPTER 9: Sleep and the Advantages of a Well-Rested Brain

179 *We also know that insomnia—a general term referring to problems maintaining sleep throughout the night*: See E. Fortier-Brochu et al. (2012), Insomnia and daytime cognitive performance: A meta-analysis, *Sleep Medicine Reviews*, 16, 83–94.

179 *The sweet spot of sleep for most people is 7 to 8 hours per night*: For a detailed discussion of this topic, see M.A. Grandner et al. (2010), Mortality associated with short sleep duration: The evidence, the possible mechanisms, the future, *Sleep Medicine Reviews*, 14, 191–203.

179 *While many people sleep in the ideal 7- to 8-hour range, over 30% of people sleep more or less*: A large study—with more than 110,000 people—looked at sleep duration across the life span: P.M. Krueger and E.M. Friedman (2009), Sleep duration in the United States: A cross-sectional population-based study, *American Journal of Epidemiology*, 169(9), 1052–1063; see also Centers for Disease Control and Prevention (2012), Short sleep duration among workers— United States, 2010. *Morbidity and Mortality Weekly Report*, 61(16), 281–285.

179 *a recent survey from the National Sleep Foundation found that 65% of American adults believe in the value of sleep*: National Sleep Foundation, 2018 Sleep in America poll, http://sleepfoundation.org.

180 *We now know that sleep appears to flush beta-amyloid from the brain*: See L. Xie et al. (2013), Sleep drives metabolite clearance from the adult brain, *Science*, 342, 373–377.

181 *This occurs by way of the glymphatic system*: See N.A. Jessen et al. (2015), The glymphatic system—A beginner's guide, *Neurochemical Research*, 40(12), 2583–2599.

181 *Some recent research nails home this point: people who report poor sleep quality*: See K.E. Sprecher et al. (2017), Poor sleep is associated with CSF biomarkers of amyloid pathology in cognitively nor-

mal adults, *Neurology*, 89, 445–453; see also K.E. Sprecher et al. (2015), Amyloid burden is associated with self-reported sleep in non-demented late middle-aged adults, *Neurobiology of Aging*, 36(9), 2568–2576.

181 *We also see that over time, beta-amyloid accumulates faster in the brains of people who report lots of daytime sleepiness:* See D.Z. Carvalho et al. (2018), Association of excessive daytime sleepiness with longitudinal β-amyloid accumulation in elderly persons without dementia, *JAMA Neurology*, 75(6), 672–680.

181 *people who sleep poorly have a higher risk of developing cognitive impairment and Alzheimer's disease:* In the largest meta-analytic study to date addressing this question, 27 studies were included, with a sample of over 69,000 people. See O.M. Bubu et al. (2017), Sleep, cognitive impairment, and Alzheimer's disease: A systematic review and meta-analysis, *Sleep*, 40(1), 1–18.

181 *Other evidence points to sleep disturbance interfering with frontal lobe functioning:* See J.S. Randolph and J.J. Randolph (2013), Modifiable lifestyle factors and cognition through midlife, in J.J. Randolph (Ed.), *Positive Neuropsychology: Evidence-Based Perspectives on Promoting Cognitive Health* (pp. 25–55), New York, NY: Springer Science+Business Media, LLC.

182 *One well-conducted study looked at the effects of restricting sleep to 4 or 6 hours per night:* See H.P.A. Van Dongen et al. (2003), The cumulative cost of additional wakefulness: Dose-response effects on neurobehavioral functions and sleep physiology from chronic sleep restriction and total sleep deprivation, *Sleep*, 2, 117–126.

183 *multiple studies have found that regularly sleeping more than 9 hours per night:* See J.S. Randolph and J.J. Randolph (2013) above.

183 *short sleeping, particularly sleeping less than 6 hours per night, has also been linked to a number of health problems:* A large review and meta-analysis looking at more than 150 studies including over 5 million people has the most definitive findings here: O. Itani et al. (2017), Short sleep duration and health outcomes: A systematic review, meta-analysis, and meta-regression, *Sleep Medicine*, 32, 246–256. A similar study assessing health effects of long sleeping was conducted by the same research group: M. Jike et al. (2018), Long sleep duration and health outcomes: A systematic review, meta-analysis and meta-regression, *Sleep Medicine Reviews*, 39, 25–36.

186 *Some research has shown that naps can improve our executive function-*

ing: See J. Mantua and R.M.C. Spencer (2017), Exploring the nap paradox: Are mid-day sleep bouts a friend or foe? *Sleep Medicine, 37*, 88–97; see also B. Faraut et al. (2017), Napping: A public health issue. From epidemiological to laboratory studies, *Sleep Medicine Reviews, 35*, 85–100.

186 *napping seems particularly helpful at clearing out adenosine*: See J. Mantua and R.M.C. Spencer (2017) above.

186 *If you're a coffee drinker, you're already familiar with the effects of adenosine*: See C.F. Reichert et al. (2016), Sleep-wake regulation and its impact on working memory performance: The role of adenosine, *Biology, 5*, 11, doi:10.3390/biology5010011.

186 *There's also evidence that napping reduces inflammation*: See B. Faraut et al. (2015), Napping reverses the salivary interleukin-6 and urinary norepinephrine changes induced by sleep restriction, *Journal of Clinical Endocrinology and Metabolism, 100*(3), E416–E426.

186 *Studies indicate that naps of less than 30 minutes*: See C.J. Hilditch et al. (2017), A review of short naps and sleep inertia: Do naps of 30 min or less really avoid sleep inertia and slow-wave sleep? *Sleep Medicine, 32*, 176–190.

187 *It also seems that napping in the afternoon*: See N. Lovato and L. Lack (2010), The effects of napping on cognitive functioning, *Progress in Brain Research, 185*, 155–166.

187 *the need to take naps more frequently can be a clear indicator of nighttime sleep problems*: See S.E. Goldman et al. (2015), Association between nighttime sleep and napping in older adults, *Sleep, 31*(5), 733–740.

187 *people who consistently nap longer than 30 minutes*: See K.-I. Jung et al. (2012), Gender differences in nighttime sleep and daytime napping as predictors of mortality in older adults: The Rancho Bernardo Study, *Sleep Medicine, 14*, 12–19.

188 *People with a distinct purpose in life*: For an example of research related to purpose in life and reduced risk of cognitive impairment, see P.A. Boyle et al. (2010), Effect of a purpose in life on risk of incident Alzheimer disease and mild cognitive impairment in community-dwelling older persons, *Archives of General Psychiatry, 67*(3), 304–310.

188 *One 4-year study looked at sleep problems and purpose in life in a group of over 4,000 people*: See E.S. Kim et al. (2015), Purpose in life and incidence of sleep disturbances, *Journal of Behavioral Medicine, 38*, 590–597.

188 *Other work has found that leading a purposeful life reduces the risk of*

sleep-related disorders: See A.D. Turner et al. (2017), Is purpose in life associated with less sleep disturbance in older adults? *Sleep Science and Practice, 1*, 14, doi:10.1186/s41606-017-0015-6.

189 *when people engage in gratitude exercises—like regularly recording what they're grateful for in a diary*: See M. Jackowska et al. (2016), The impact of a brief gratitude intervention on subjective well-being, biology and sleep, *Journal of Health Psychology, 21*(10), 2207–2217, doi:10.1177/1359105315572455.

189 *While it's unclear why showing gratitude improves sleep quality, there's some evidence that people have fewer troubling thoughts at night*: See A.M. Wood et al. (2009), Gratitude influences sleep through the mechanism of pre-sleep cognitions, *Journal of Psychosomatic Research, 66*, 43–48.

190 *Some structures in the brain, including the memory-critical hippocampus, are particularly vulnerable*: See R.S. Bucks et al. (2017), Reviewing the relationship between OSA and cognition: Where do we go from here? *Respirology, 22*, 1253–1261.

190 *But for those who do, concentration and memory are commonly affected*: For recent studies examining cognitive problems in individuals with sleep apnea, see M. Olaithe et al. (2018), Cognitive deficits in obstructive sleep apnea: Insights from a meta-review and comparison with deficits observed in COPD, insomnia, and sleep deprivation, *Sleep Medicine Reviews, 38*, 39–49; Y. Leng et al. (2017), Association of sleep-disordered breathing with cognitive function and risk of cognitive impairment: A systematic review and meta-analysis, *JAMA Neurology, 74*(10), 1237–1245; and R.S. Bucks et al. (2017) above.

191 *Sleep researchers have also discovered that people with sleep-disordered breathing experience cognitive changes (including dementia) earlier than others*: See R.S. Osorio et al. (2015), Sleep-disordered breathing advances cognitive decline in the elderly, *Neurology, 84*, 1964–1971.

191 *People consistently using CPAP show improved thinking skills in multiple areas*: For an example of a study showing improved executive functioning with CPAP treatment, see M. Olaithe and R.S. Bucks (2013), Executive dysfunction in OSA before and after treatment: A meta-analysis, *Sleep, 36*(9), 1297–1305.

192 *Teen drivers in school districts with earlier start times*: For the most comprehensive study to date in this area, see K. Wahlstrom et al. (2014), *Examining the Impact of Later School Start Times on the Health*

and Academic Performance of High School Students: A Multi-Site Study, St. Paul, MN: Center for Applied Research and Educational Improvement, University of Minnesota; see also J.A. Owens et al. (2010), Impact of delaying school start time on adolescent sleep, mood, and behavior, *Archives of Pediatrics and Adolescent Medicine*, 164(7), 608–614.

192 *This could be due to the negative effects of sleep deprivation on information processing speed*: See M. Cohen-Zion et al. (2016), Effects of partial sleep deprivation on information processing speed in adolescence, *Journal of the International Neuropsychological Society*, 22, 1–11.

192 *research has also shown that the later schools begin classes, the more sleep students get*: For a recent study in this regard that used wrist activity monitors to accurately gauge sleep and wake time, see G.P. Dunster et al. (2018), Sleep*more* in Seattle: Later school start times are associated with more sleep and better performance in high school students, *Science Advances*, 4, eaau6200.

192 *There's also evidence that kids in delayed-start districts have better interactions*: For a recent example of reduced disciplinary problems when a 45-minute delay was implemented, see P.V. Thacher and S.V. Onyper (2016), Longitudinal outcomes of start time delay on sleep, behavior, and achievement in high school, *Sleep*, *39*(2), 271–281.

CHAPTER 10: Mellowing the Stressed-Out Brain

199 *Take the classic Yerkes–Dodson law of stress*: For the original article, see R.M. Yerkes and J.D. Dodson (1908), The relation of strength of stimulus to rapidity of habit-formation, *Journal of Comparative Neurology and Psychology*, 18, 459–482; for a more recent discussion of how this law has been considered over the years, see K.H. Teigen (1994), Yerkes-Dodson: A law for all seasons, *Theory & Psychology*, 4(4), 525–547.

200 *there's a whimsical but descriptive term coined by psychologist Daniel Goleman*: In his book on emotional intelligence, Goleman describes this concept in some detail. See D. Goleman (2005), *Emotional Intelligence: Why It Can Matter More than IQ*, New York, NY: Bantam Books.

200 *some research has shown that the connection between the amygdala and the frontal lobes is essentially severed*: See H. Jovanovic et al. (2011),

Chronic stress is linked to 5-HT1A receptor changes and functional disintegration of the limbic networks, *NeuroImage*, *55*, 1178–1188.

202 *too much cortisol can negatively affect multiple cognitive skills*: As one example of this research, see C.E. Franz et al. (2011), Cross-sectional and 35-year longitudinal assessment of salivary cortisol and cognitive functioning: The Vietnam Era Twin Study of Aging, *Psychoneuroendocrinology*, *36*, 1040–1052.

202 *The hippocampus is one of the areas most affected by stress*: See M.-K. Sun and D.L. Alkon (2014), Stress: Perspectives on its impact on cognition and pharmacological treatment, *Behavioural Pharmacology*, *25*, 410–424; see also H. Jovanovic et al. (2011) above.

202 *The hippocampus is particularly vulnerable because it has lots of glucocorticoid receptors*: J.C. Pruessner et al. (2005), Self-esteem, locus of control, hippocampal volume, and cortisol regulation in young and old adulthood, *NeuroImage*, *28*, 815–826.

202 *One of the key executive functions we rely on in daily life—mental flexibility*: See G.S. Shields et al. (2016), The effects of acute stress on core executive functions: A meta-analysis and comparison with cortisol, *Neuroscience and Biobehavioral Reviews*, *68*, 651–668.

203 *One study had people engage in two activities that many people consider stressful*: See J.K. Alexander et al. (2007), Beta-adrenergic modulation of cognitive flexibility during stress, *Journal of Cognitive Neuroscience*, *19*(3), 468–478.

204 *Some research has found that stress interferes with remembering information for brief periods*: M. Luethi et al. (2009), Stress effects on working memory, explicit memory, and implicit memory for neutral and emotional stimuli in healthy men, *Frontiers in Behavioral Neuroscience*, *2*, article 5, doi:10.3389/neuro.08.005.2008.

205 *problems can also take the form of reacting more impulsively when we're under stress* See A.F.T. Arnsten (2009), Stress signaling pathways that impair prefrontal cortex structure and function, *Nature Reviews Neuroscience*, *10*(6), 410–422.

205 *It seems that levels of two neurotransmitters—dopamine and norepinephrine—help determine the extent to which stress affects our cognitive abilities*: See A.F.T. Arnsten (2009) above.

205 *One study considered a situation that many of us would describe as*

pretty stressful: preparing for a major exam: See C. Liston et al. (2009), Psychosocial stress reversibly disrupts prefrontal processing and attentional control, *Proceedings of the National Academy of Sciences USA*, 106(3), 912–917.

207 *Some research has looked at the frequency of stressful life events across a few months*: See S.A. Papagni et al. (2011), Effects of stressful life events on human brain structure: A longitudinal voxel-based morphometry study, *Stress*, 14(2), 227–232.

207 *a longitudinal study considered the effects of stress on the brain over a 20-year period*: P.J. Gianaros et al. (2007), Prospective reports of chronic life stress predict decreased grey matter volume in the hippocampus, *NeuroImage*, 35, 795–803.

208 *particularly regarding the detrimental effects of chronic stress on multiple areas within the prefrontal cortex*: See E.B. Ansell et al. (2012), Cumulative adversity and smaller gray matter volume in medial prefrontal, anterior cingulate, and insula regions, *Biological Psychiatry*, 72, 57–64.

208 *those reporting high levels of stress over the course of a decade*: See R.S. Wilson et al. (2007), Chronic distress and incidence of mild cognitive impairment, *Neurology*, 68, 2085–2092.

208 *one study looked at individuals who were within 1.5 miles of the 9/11 World Trade Center terrorist attack*: See B.L. Ganzel et al. (2008), Resilience after 9/11: Multimodal neuroimaging evidence for stress-related change in the healthy adult brain, *NeuroImage*, 40, 788–795.

211 *Even attending to a specific sense—part of what's called effortless awareness*: One example of a study that used this style of mindfulness in the context of brain activity is by R. van Lutterveld et al. (2017), Meditation is associated with increased brain network integration, *NeuroImage*, 158, 18–25.

212 *meditation, broadly speaking, helps promote richer connections*: See K.C.R. Fox et al. (2014), Is meditation associated with altered brain structure? A systematic review and meta-analysis of morphometric neuroimaging in meditation practitioners, *Neuroscience and Biobehavioral Reviews*, 43, 48–73.

212 *And we know that certain types of mindfulness—such as simply labeling our emotional states*: See J.D. Creswell et al. (2007), Neural correlates of dispositional mindfulness during affect labeling, *Psychosomatic Medicine*, 69, 560–565.

212 *One study had people engage in MBSR for 8 weeks*: See B.K. Holzel et al. (2011), Mindfulness practice leads to increases in regional brain gray matter density, *Psychiatry Research: Neuroimaging, 191,* 36–43.

213 *expert meditators showed more integration throughout the brain*: See R. van Lutterveld et al. (2017) above.

213 *meditators tend to be effective at maintaining their focus for extended periods*: See P. Sedlmeier et al. (2012), The psychological effects of meditation: A meta-analysis, *Psychological Bulletin, 1386,* 1139–1171.

213 *One recent study examined people who had consistently practiced yoga for 3 or more years*: See N.P. Goethe et al. (2018), Differences in brain structure and function among yoga practitioners and controls, *Frontiers in Integrative Neuroscience, 12,* 26.

214 *yoga practice is linked to benefits for cognitive skills*: See N.P. Gothe et al. (2015), Yoga and cognition: A meta-analysis of chronic and acute effects, *Psychosomatic Medicine, 77,* 784–797.

214 *A powerful study a few years ago asked a group of college students to determine their top two personal values*: See D.K. Sherman et al. (2009), Psychological vulnerability and stress: The effects of self-affirmation on sympathetic nervous system responses to naturalistic stressors, *Health Psychology, 28*(5), 554–562.

215 *people were asked to write in a diary about things they were grateful for*: See M. Jackowska et al. (2016), The impact of a brief gratitude intervention on subjective well-being, biology and sleep. *Journal of Health Psychology, 21*(10), 2207–2217, doi:10.1177/1359105315572455.

216 *People who are more physically active (either through aerobic activity or weight training) tend to report better emotional functioning*: Two large recent studies further clarified the benefits of exercise on mental health. See S. Chekroud et al. (2018), Association between physical exercise and mental health in 1.2 million individuals in the USA between 2011 and 2015: A cross-sectional study, *Lancet Psychiatry, 5,* 739–746; and B.R. Gordon et al. (2018), Association of efficacy of resistance exercise training with depressive symptoms: Meta-analysis and meta-regression analysis of randomized clinical trials, *JAMA Psychiatry, 75*(6), 566–576.

CHAPTER 11: Do Medical Problems and Smoking Affect How My Brain Works?

223 *It turns out that diabetes can lead to problems with a few key thinking skills*: See P. Palta et al. (2014), Magnitude of cognitive dysfunction in adults with type 2 diabetes: A meta-analysis of six cognitive domains and the most frequently reported neuropsychological tests within domains, *Journal of the International Neuropsycholog-ical Society, 20*, 278–291; see also E. Pelimanni and M. Jehkonen (2019), Type 2 diabetes and cognitive functions in middle age: A meta-analysis, *Journal of the International Neuropsychological Society, 25*(2), 215–229.

223 *people with diabetes tend to show increased difficulties with conversa-tional word-finding too*: See P. Palta et al. (2018), Diabetes and cog-nitive decline in older adults: The Ginkgo Evaluation of Memory Study, *Journals of Gerontology, Series A: Biological Sciences and Med-ical Sciences, 73*(1), 123–130.

223 *One recent study followed thousands of diabetics over the course of about 10 years*: See F. Zheng et al. (2018), HbA1c, diabetes and cognitive decline: The English Longitudinal Study of Ageing, *Diabetologica, 61*, 839–848.

224 *Type 1 diabetes—most often diagnosed in kids*: See C.M. Ryan et al. (2016), Neurocognitive consequences of diabetes, *American Psychol-ogist, 71*(7), 563–576.

224 *Scientists believe that these changes occur in a few different ways*: For an excellent review of this topic, see Ryan et al. (2016) above.

225 *some brain regions can be smaller in diabetics*: See C. Moran et al. (2013), Brain atrophy in type 2 diabetes: Regional distribution and influence on cognition, *Diabetes Care, 36*, 4036–4042.

225 *There's also evidence of weaker connections between different brain struc-tures*: See Y.D. Reijmer et al. (2013), Disruption of the cerebral white matter network is related to slowing of information pro-cessing speed in patients with type 2 diabetes, *Diabetes, 62*, 2112–2115. Another study looked at similar issues: C. Qiu et al. (2014), Diabetes, markers of brain pathology and cognitive function: The Age, Gene/Environment Susceptibility-Reykjavik Study, *Annals of Neurology, 75*, 138–146.

225 *Notably, diabetes is a risk factor for dementia, particularly if diagnosed in midlife*: See A.M. Tolppanen et al. (2012), Midlife vascular risk factors and Alzheimer's disease: Evidence from epidemiological studies, *Journal of Alzheimer's Disease, 32*, 531–540.

225 *There's some related research indicating that adhering to the MeDi might also prevent type 2 diabetes:* See L. Schwingshackl et al. (2014), Adherence to a Mediterranean diet and risk of diabetes: A systematic review and meta-analysis, *Public Health Nutrition,* 18(7), 1292–1299.

225 *And gaining better control over blood sugar levels is linked to greater overall brain size and improved cognition:* See L.L. Launer et al. (2011), Effects of randomization to intensive glucose lowering on brain structure and function in type 2 diabetes ACCORD Memory in Diabetes Study, *Lancet Neurology,* 10(11), 969–977; and C.M. Ryan et al. (2006), Improving metabolic control leads to better working memory in adults with type 2 diabetes, *Diabetes Care,* 29, 345–351.

225 *There's the added benefit of improving general health with increased physical fitness:* A large recent study found a significantly lower risk of conditions such as diabetes, cancer, and lung disease in people who engaged in modest levels of physical activity; see A. Marques et al. (2019), Cross-sectional and prospective relationship between low-to-moderate-intensity physical activity and chronic diseases in older adults from 13 European countries, *Journal of Aging and Physical Activity,* 27, 93–101.

226 *a recent survey found that about a third of U.S. adults have high blood pressure:* A recent survey on this topic includes many details about hypertension in the United States; see C.D. Fryar et al. (2017), *Hypertension Prevalence and Control among Adults: United States, 2015–2016,* NCHS Data Brief, no. 289, Hyattsville, MD: National Center for Health Statistics.

226 *although it also has been linked to mild cognitive impairment:* A variety of studies have examined related issues. See T.W. Budford (2016), Hypertension and aging, *Ageing Research Reviews,* 26, 96–111; see also L.J. Launer et al. (2000), Midlife blood pressure and dementia: The Honolulu-Asia aging study, *Neurobiology of Aging,* 21(1), 49–55.

226 *Hypertension is known to diminish multiple cognitive skills:* A recent meta-analysis found that after accounting for other factors such as diabetes and high cholesterol, hypertension affected memory and global cognitive ability. See K.A. Gifford et al. (2013), Blood pressure and cognition among older adults: A meta-analysis, *Archives of Clinical Neuropsychology,* 28, 649–664.

226 *Some recent research found that hypertension was linked to a 65% increased risk of dementia:* See P. Gilsanz et al. (2017), Female sex, early-onset hypertension, and risk of dementia, *Neurology,* 89, 1886–1893.

227 *There's also evidence that midlife high blood pressure can lead to dementia in men*: See L.J. Launer et al. (2000) above.

227 *successfully reducing blood pressure can minimize the risk of cognitive problems*: See The SPRINT MIND Investigators (2019), Effect of intensive vs. standard blood pressure control on probable dementia: A randomized clinical trial, *JAMA*, *321*(6), 553–561, doi:10.1001/jama.2018.21442.

227 *One recent study specifically looked at how exercise affected cognition in people with cardiovascular problems*: See J.A. Blumenthal et al. (2019), Lifestyle and neurocognition in older adults with cognitive impairments, *Neurology*, *92*, e1–e12, doi:10.1212/WNL.0000000000006784.

227 *Keep in mind that some earlier research has found specific cognitive benefits from the DASH diet*: One study found that the DASH diet in isolation improved processing speed, although combined with exercise, there were more benefits for the brain. See P.J. Smith et al. (2010), Effects of the Dietary Approaches to Stop Hypertension diet, exercise, and caloric restriction on neurocognition in overweight adults with high blood pressure, *Hypertension*, *55*, 1331–1338; see also H. Wengreen et al. (2013), Prospective study of Dietary Approaches to Stop Hypertension and Mediterranean-style dietary patterns and age-related cognitive changes: The Cache County study on memory, health and aging, *American Journal of Clinical Nutrition*, *98*, 1263–1271.

228 *At this point, more than one third of U.S. adults are obese*: See C.L. Ogden et al. (2015), *Prevalence of Obesity among Adults and Youth: United States, 2011–2014*, NCHS Data Brief, no. 219, Hyattsville, MD, National Center for Health Statistics.

228 *having no health issues other than being overweight is linked to less brain volume*: See C.A. Raji et al. (2010), Brain structure and obesity, *Human Brain Mapping*, *31*(3), 353–364.

228 *Some research has found that being overweight can interfere with your ability to make decisions, plan, and think flexibly*: See S. Fitzpatrick et al. (2013), Systematic review: Are overweight and obese individuals impaired on behavioural tasks of executive functioning? *Neuropsychology Review*, *23*, 138–156.

228 *being obese in midlife significantly increases one's chances of cognitive problems many years down the road*: See D.S. Knopman et al. (2018), Midlife vascular risk factors and midlife cognitive status in rela-

tion to prevalence of mild cognitive impairment and dementia in later life: The Atherosclerosis Risk in Communities Study, *Alzheimer's & Dementia*, 14, 1406–1415; see also W.L. Xu et al. (2011), Midlife overweight and obesity increase late-life dementia risk, *Neurology*, 76, 1568–1574.

229 *Adding insult to injury, high total cholesterol levels*: See KJ Anstey et al. (2008), Cholesterol as a risk factor for dementia and cognitive decline: A systematic review of prospective studies with meta-analysis, *American Journal of Geriatric Psychiatry*, 16(5), 343–354.

229 *Some science indicates that becoming more physically active may be more important for your health*: See V.W. Barry et al. (2014), Fitness vs. fatness on all-cause mortality: A meta-analysis, *Progress in Cardiovascular Diseases*, 56, 382–390.

229 *There's also evidence that reducing your weight can lead to improved thinking skills*: See S. Masi et al. (2018), Patterns of adiposity, vascular phenotypes, and cognitive function in the 1946 British Birth Cohort, *BMC Medicine*, 16, 75.

229 *a Mediterranean-style diet can help with weight reduction*: See K. Esposito et al. (2004), Effect of a Mediterranean-style diet on endothelial dysfunction and markers of vascular inflammation in the metabolic syndrome, *JAMA*, 292(12), 1440–1446; see also A. Jula et al. (2002), Effects of diet and simvastatin on serum lipids, insulin, and antioxidants in hypercholesterolemic men, *JAMA*, 287(5), 598–605.

230 *While there have been recent calls to reduce nicotine levels in cigarettes*: See B.J. Apelberg et al. (2018), Potential public health effects of reducing nicotine levels in cigarettes in the United States, *New England Journal of Medicine*, 378(18), 1725–1733.

230 *Smoking appears to affect the brain on levels large and small*: See T.C. Durazzo et al. (2010), Chronic cigarette smoking: Implications for neurocognition and brain neurobiology, *International Journal of Environmental Research and Public Health*, 7, 3760–3791; see also J. Gallinat et al. (2006), Smoking and structural brain deficits: A volumetric MR investigation, *European Journal of Neuroscience*, 24, 1744–1750.

230 *smoking can impair our efforts to learn and remember new information we hear or see*: See T.C. Durazzo et al. (2012), A comprehensive assessment of neurocognition in middle-aged chronic cigarette

smokers, *Drug and Alcohol Dependence, 122,* 105–111; and T.C. Durazzo et al. (2010) above.

231   *Multiple studies have also shown that smokers' thinking skills decline faster over time:* See A.C.J. Nooyens et al. (2008), Smoking and cognitive decline among middle-aged men and women: The Doetinchem Cohort Study, *American Journal of Public Health,* 98(12), 2244–2250; see also S. Sabia et al. (2012), Impact of smoking on cognitive decline in early old age: The Whitehall II Cohort Study, *Archives of General Psychiatry,* 69(6), 627–635.

231   *Experts agree that as a strategy to prevent different forms of dementia, quitting smoking definitely counts:* See K. Deckers et al. (2014), Target risk factors for dementia prevention: A systematic review and Delphi consensus study on the evidence from observational studies, *International Journal of Geriatric Psychiatry,* 30, 234–246.

231   *one large study followed nearly 9,000 people in their early forties for about 25 years:* See R.A. Whitmer et al. (2005), Midlife cardiovascular risk factors and risk of dementia in late life, *Neurology,* 64, 277–281.

231   *Other scientists have proposed that millions of individuals worldwide could have potentially avoided Alzheimer's disease:* See D.E Barnes and K. Yaffe (2011), The projected impact of risk factor reduction on Alzheimer's disease prevalence, *Lancet Neurology,* 10(9), 819–828.

231   *The science indicates that kicking the habit can result in memory and executive function gains:* See Nooyens et al. (2008) above.

231   *After about 10 years of not smoking, ex-smokers show expected age-related cognitive changes at about the same rate:* See Sabia et al. (2012) above.

CHAPTER 12: Locking in Brain-Healthy Lifestyle Changes

241   *About 50% of people who intend to change their behavior fail to do so:* For a detailed review of what's called the *intention–behavior gap,* see P. Sheeran (2002), Intention-behavior relations: A conceptual and empirical review, *European Review of Social Psychology,* 12(1), 1–36.

241   *A group of young adults was asked to consider a type of behavior they wanted to add to their lives:* See P. Lally et al. (2010), How are habits formed: Modelling habit formation in the real world, *European Journal of Social Psychology,* 40, 998–1009.

242   *One interesting study specifically looked at how long it takes to develop a new exercise routine:* See C.J. Armitage (2005), Can the theory

of planned behavior predict the maintenance of physical activity? *Health Psychology, 24(3),* 235–245.

243 *When we consider how habits are formed, research points to four key steps:* For a great summary of the research on promoting new habits, see P. Lally and B. Gardner (2013), Promoting habit formation, *Health Psychology Review, 7(1),* S137–S158.

244 *From a brain-based standpoint, something becomes habitual when you no longer have to think deliberately about doing it:* For a detailed technical discussion of the neuroanatomy of habits, see H.H. Yin and B.J. Knowlton (2006), The role of the basal ganglia in habit formation, *Nature Reviews Neuroscience, 7,* 464–476.

245 *One way to increase the chances of successfully incorporating a new lifestyle change is to have a built-in reminder:* See Lally and Gardener (2013) above.

246 *enjoying a new activity clearly increases the chances of us continuing to do it:* See P. Van Cappellen et al. (2018), Positive affective processes underlie positive health behavior change, *Psychology and Health, 33(1),* 77–97.

247 *One study looked at factors linked to how well people were able to improve their diets:* This was a large meta-regression study that allowed for an analysis of specific strategies that affect nutrition and physical activity. See S. Michie et al. (2009), Effective techniques in healthy eating and physical activity interventions: A meta-regression, *Health Psychology, 28(6),* 690–701.

248 *research shows that we're better at achieving our goals when we've let others know what they are:* For an example of related research, see B. Harkin et al. (2016), Does monitoring goal progress promote goal attainment? A meta-analysis of the experimental evidence, *Psychological Bulletin, 142(2),* 198–229.

248 *physically record how we're doing with our goals:* See B. Harkin et al. (2016) above.

250 *What's referred to as vigilant monitoring:* See J.M. Quinn et al. (2010): Can't control yourself? Monitor those bad habits, *Personality and Social Psychology Bulletin, 36(4),* 499–511.

INDEX

Note: Italicized page locators refer to figures.